From Hypertension to Heart Failure

GW00602694

With Compliments

F. Hoffmann-La Roche Ltd

Springer

Berlin
Heidelberg
New York
Barcelona
Budapest
Hong Kong
London
Milan
Paris
Santa Clara
Singapore
Tokyo

M. Böhm   J. H. Laragh   M. Zehender (Eds.)

From Hypertension to Heart Failure

With 36 Figures

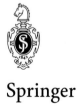

Springer

Professor Dr. med. MICHAEL BÖHM
Klinik III für Innere Medizin der Universität Köln
Josef-Stelzmann-Straße 9, 50924 Köln, Germany

Professor JOHN H. LARAGH
The New York Hospital, Cornell Medical Center
526 East 68th Street, New York, NY 10021, USA

Priv.-Doz. Dr. med. MANFRED ZEHENDER
Med. Universitätsklinik und Poliklinik
Abteilung Innere Medizin III
Hugstetterstraße 55, 79106 Freiburg, Germany

ISBN 3-540-63542-4 Springer-Verlag Berlin Heidelberg New York

Library of Congress Cataloging-in-Publication Data
From hypertension to heart failure / M. Böhm, J. H. Laragh, M. Zehender
(eds.). p. cm. Includes bibliographical references and index.
ISBN 3-540-63542-4 (pbk. : alk. paper)
1. Heart failure. 2. Hypertension. 3. Coronary heart disease. 4. Adrenergic beta blockers.
I. Böhm, M. (Michael), 1958– . II. Laragh, John H., 1924– .
[DNLM: 1. Heart Failure, Congestive–drug therapy. 2. Heart Failure, Congestive–physio-
pathology. 3. Coronary Disease–drug therapy. 4. Hypertension–drug therapy. 5. Adrenergic
beta-Antagonists–therapeutic use. WG 370 F931 1998]
RC685.C53.F76 1998   616.1'29–dc21   DNLM/DLC
for Library of Congress   98-17988   CIP

© Springer-Verlag Berlin · Heidelberg 1998
Printed in Germany

Cover-Design: Design & Production GmbH, Heidelberg
Typesetting: K+V Fotosatz GmbH, Beerfelden

SPIN 10736239   18/3111-5 4 3 2 1 – Printed on acid-free paper

Preface

Arterial hypertension, coronary heart disease and heart failure are the commonest cardiovascular conditions to present in clinical practice. Over the past few years it has become increasingly clear that they are closely and causally interrelated and that their relationship can have a significant bearing on prognosis. Epidemiological studies have shown that arterial hypertension is one of the most important risk factors for developing heart failure. Only one in four patients with hypertension is adequately managed, and in 50% of cases, the hypertension has not been recognised or treated. Patients with pre-existing hypertension who go on to suffer an acute myocardial infarction have usually not previously had typical angina symptoms, the infarct territory is larger, life threatening arrhythmias are commoner and hence in-hospital mortality and long-term prognosis are markedly worse. The presence of raised blood pressure in the post-infarct phase doubles the risk of manifest heart failure.

The close relationship between hypertension, coronary heart disease and heart failure makes the choice of therapeutic strategy particularly important. Agents and classes of agents that have prognostic value in all three conditions should be considered first, as synergy might result in additional benefits. In such patients, this sort of therapeutic decision-making might have further advantages. The use of these agents may prevent complications which are not yet clinically obvious (such as heart failure). With medication that tackles all three disease components, it might also be possible to create more comprehensive patient-friendly treatment regimen with an overall reduction in drug use, better compliance and fewer side-effects. In addition, the economic importance of using a single agent should not be underestimated.

Beta blockers have been in clinical use since the 1970s, and are experiencing something of a renaissance as novel therapeutic strategies in certain situations. In the treatment of hypertension, it is already clear that effective lowering of blood pressure in the long-term, prognostic benefit for left ventricular hypertrophy and improvement in overall prognosis only occurs if vasodilatation is accompanied by a sympatholytic component with autonomic inhibition. Of particular interest are those recently introduced beta blockers that offer an additional vasodilating component.

Beta blockers have a secure position in the treatment of coronary heart disease, as many controlled studies have shown that they improve prognosis after myocardial infarction. It has only recently become apparent, however, that this class of agents can also be beneficial in unstable angina and in acute myocardial infarction, providing there are no contraindications to treatment. This increasingly positive view of beta blockers applies to their effects on sudden cardiac death, especially in patients with coronary artery disease, where class I and III anti-arrhythmic drugs can have significant side effects. Beta blockers do not act by affecting the frequency of ventricular arrhythmias, instead they have an overall protective action, mostly through increasing the fibrillation threshold and beneficial effects on arrhythmogenic cofactors (such as ischaemia or the autonomic system) and thus reduce the sudden cardiac death rates by 25%.

A similar novel strategy is to use beta blockers in patients with latent or manifest heart failure. Data on their potential benefits have been available for many years from the end of the 1960s, but persuasive results have only relatively recently emerged from four large trials tackling this question. In particular, the latest generation of beta blockers with vasodilating properties appear to have a convincing benefit on mortality in patients with heart failure. Carvedilol is one such drug available in this class. It is now licensed for this condition and this turns the previous paradigm of heart failure being a contraindication for beta blockers upside down.

The aim of this book is to provide an overview of the wide-ranging therapeutic uses of beta blockers, particularly in common diseases which are prognostically related, including arterial hypertension, coronary heart disease and heart failure. The book will concentrate on the usefulness of the newest generation of vasodilating beta blockers, typified by carvedilol, with the main emphasis on describing this compound, which has received particular attention in the field.

M. Böhm
J.H. Laragh
March 1998   M. Zehender

Contents

List of Contributors

Böhm, Michael, Prof. Dr., Universität zu Köln,
Klinik III für Innere Medizin, Joseph-Stelzmann-Straße 9,
D-50924 Köln

Christ, Michael, Dr., Ruprecht-Karls-Universität Heidelberg,
Fakultät für Klinische Medizin Mannheim,
Institut für Klinische Pharmakologie, Theodor-Kutzer-Ufer,
D-68167 Mannheim

Flesch, M., Dr., Universität zu Köln,
Klinik III für Innere Medizin, Joseph-Stelzmann-Straße 9,
D-50924 Köln

Franz, Ingomar-W., Prof. Dr.,
Rehabilitationsklinik Wehrawald, Schwarzenbacher Straße 3,
D-79682 Todtmoos

Haberl, Ralph, Priv.-Doz. Dr.,
Medizinische Klinik I der Universität, Klinikum Großhadern,
Marchionistraße 15, D-81377 München

Himmelmann, Anders, Prof. Dr.,
Sahlgrenska University Hospital,
Department of Clinical Pharmacology, S-41345 Göteborg

Kannel, W.B., MD, MPH,
Boston University School of Medicine,
BU-Framingham Study, 5 Thurber Street, Framingham,
Massachusetts 01760, USA

Lahiri, Avijit, MB, BS, MSc, MRCP, FACC, FESC,
Northwick Park Hospital and Clinical Research Center,
Watford Road, Harrow Middlesex HA1 3UJ, UK

Lahiri, Nayana, MD, St. George's Hospital, Medical School,
London, United Kingdom

Loo, van de, Andreas, Dr.,
Klinikum der Albert-Ludwigs-Universität,
Abteilung Innere Medizin III, Hugstetter Straße 55,
D-79106 Freiburg

Maack, Christoph, Dr., Universität zu Köln,
Klinik III für Innere Medizin, Joseph-Stelzmann-Straße 9,
D-50924 Köln

Hartmann, D., Dr., Universität zu Köln,
Klinik III für Innere Medizin, Joseph-Stelzmann-Straße 9,
D-50924 Köln

Poole-Wilson, Philip A., MD, FRCP, FACC, FESC,
National Heart and Lung Institute,
Department of Cardiac Medicine, Dovehouse Street,
London SW3 6LY, UK

Rohrer, Daniel, PhD, Stanford University Medical Center,
Department of Molecular and Cellular Physiology,
Beckmann Center 159, Stanford, CA 94305-5345, USA

Schnabel, Petra, Dr., Universität zu Köln,
Klinik III für Innere Medizin, Joseph-Stelzmann-Straße 9,
D-50924 Köln

Soman, Prem, MD,
Northwick Park Hospital and Clinical Research Center,
Watford Road, Harrow Middlesex HA1 3UJ, UK

Stäblein, A., Dr., Universität zu Köln,
Klinik III für Innere Medizin, Joseph-Stelzmann-Straße 9,
D-50924 Köln

Steinbeck, Gerhard, Prof. Dr.,
Medizinische Klinik I der Universität, Klinikum Großhadern,
Marchioninistraße 15, D-81377 München

Wehling, M., Prof. Dr.,
Ruprecht-Karls-Universität Heidelberg,
Fakultät für Klinische Medizin Mannheim,
Institut für Klinische Pharmakologie, Theodor-Kutzer-Ufer,
D-68167 Mannheim

PART I

Introduction

CHAPTER 1

Epidemiologic Insights into Progression from Hypertension to Heart Failure

W. B. Kannel

Review of national vital and health statistics and the epidemiology of cardiac failure indicates that it is a common end-stage of heart disease and a major burden on individuals and the health care systems of many countries. Morbidity and mortality attributed to it are high, survival is poor and treatment is inadequate. Heart failure ranks high in causes of hospitalizations in the US following childbirth, pneumonia, psychosis and fractures, and it is the leading diagnosis for hospitalizations of patients over age 65 years [1]. The hospitalization rate for heart failure for persons aged 45–64 years increased from 8.2 per 10000 in 1971 to 33.8 per 10000 in 1994. The continued rise in the prevalence of this condition over recent decades and its persistent high mortality rate contrasts with observed major mortality reductions from other cardiovascular events [2, 3]. These trends have made heart failure a major problem with a profound economic impact on the health care system. It is estimated that 4.8 million Americans have heart failure, 400000 developing it yearly. In 1994 there were nearly 3 million office visits for heart failure [2, 3].

Prevention and control of identified predisposing conditions have the greatest potential for ameliorating this ominous public health problem. Detection and control of hypertension and myocardial infarction, the two conditions that account for most of the heart failure in the general population, have proved to be effective against heart failure but are not fully implemented. Although treatment of hypertension and coronary disease has been actively promoted, it is estimated that 45% of patients with hypertension do not have their blood pressure adequately controlled [2, 3] Similarly, use of beta-blockers, aspirin, ACE inhibitors and thrombolytic therapy to prevent recurrences, and limit damage from myocardial infarction, is often suboptimal [2, 3]. The best prospect for curbing this major public health problem is to deal with it in evolution and correct the maladaptive process it provokes before it becomes clinically overt.

Hypertension is a recognized dominant precursor of heart failure [4, 5]. Among the major conditions predisposing to heart failure-including myocardial infarction [5–7], diabetes [8], valvular heart disease [9], left ventricular hypertrophy [10] and the cardiomyopathies – hypertension has the highest attributable risk in the general population [4, 5, 11]. Trials of the efficacy of treating hypertension have documented the benefits of treatment, but have provided little insight into the progression from asymptomatic elevation of blood pressure to overt cardiac failure. Population studies such as that at Framingham were able to examine the relationship of hypertension to the occurrence of heart failure in a population setting with a comprehensive long-term follow-up, so that the evolution from presymptomatic hypertension to overt left ventricular dysfunction can be examined and the conditions influencing the progression to cardiac failure can be identified and their impact quantified. This is important because hypertension and coronary heart disease are the chief causes of congestive heart failure in affluent countries and a reduction in morbidity and mortality from this scourge requires epidemiologic insights pointing to appropriate preventive measures likely to be effective.

Hypertensive Risk

The chief risk factors that contribute to the development of heart failure in the general population have been identified [5, 6, 10]. In particular, the Framingham study has provided data on the role of hypertension in the past [4] and more recently in 5143 hypertensive study participants followed for 20 years for the development of hypertensive heart failure. During the period of follow-up of these subjects aged 40–89 years, with blood pressures of at least 140/90 mmHg, 392 developed new onset of heart failure [12]. Adjusting for age and other associated risk factors, the hazard of developing heart failure in those subjects with hypertension was twice that of normotensive men and three times that of normoten-

Table 1. Hazard ratios and attributable risks for conditions predisposing to heart failure; Framingham study subjects 40–89 years of age

Condition	Sex	Hazard ratio	% Prevalence	% Attributable
High blood pressure	M	2.07	60	39
	F	3.35	62	59
Myocardial Infarction	M	6.34	10	34
	F	6.01	3	13
Angina	M	1.43	11	5
	F	1.68	9	5
Diabetes	M	1.82	8	6
	F	3.73	5	12
Left ventricular	M	2.19	4	4
hypertropy	F	2.85	3	5
Valvular heart disease	M	2.47	5	7
	F	2.13	8	8

All estimates are statistically significant.

sive women. In all, 91% of heart failure was preceded by some degree of blood pressure elevation [12]. Because some degree of hypertension was present in 60% of the population sample, hypertension had a high attributable risk, even exceeding that of myocardial infarction, which had a much higher risk ratio, increasing risk six fold (Table 1). Hypertension accounted for 39% and 59% of heart failure cases in men and women, respectively, whereas myocardial infarction, with a prevalence of only 3%–10%, had an attributable risk of 13%–34% (Table 1).

Thus, hypertension is a very prevalent condition in the general population that predisposes to all the major atherosclerotic cardiovascular disease outcomes including coronary heart disease, stroke, and peripheral artery disease, but with risk ratios that are greatest for cardiac failure (Table 2). Risk of failure increases in a continuous graded fashion with the severity of the hypertension and even moderate elevations of blood pressure imposing a substantial risk [12]. The average blood pressure preceding hypertensive heart failure in the Framingham study was only 150/80 mmHg (Table 3). The impact of systolic blood pressure exceeds that of diastolic pressure in both sexes, and even isolated systolic hypertension is hazardous at all ages, including old age. Isolated

Table 2. Risk of cardiovascular events in hypertensive subjects aged 35–64 years; 36-year follow-up of Framingham study

Cardiovascular events	Age-adjusted biennial rate/1000		Age-adjusted risk ratio		Excess risk per 1000	
	Men	Women	Men	Women	Men	Women
Coronary heart disease	45	21	2.0	2.2	23	12
Stroke	12	6	3.8	2.6	9	4
Periperal artery disease	10	7	2.0	3.7	5	5
Heart failure	14	6	4.0	3.0	10	4

All estimates are significant at $p<0.0001$.

Table 3. Conditions associated with hypertension progressing to heart failure; Framingham study of subjects aged 40–89 years (from [12])

Conditions	Men	Women
Systolic blood pressure	149	150
Diastolic blood pressure	81	77
Stage 1 hypertension [%]	24	18
Stage 2 or greater [%]	76	82
Myocardial infarction [%]	52	34
Angina pectoris [%]	36	35
Angina without M. I. [%]	12	21
Diabetes [%]	24	28
Left ventricular hypertrophy [%]	21	23
Valvular heart disease [%]	24	33

systolic blood pressure elevation is associated with a high pulse pressure, and risk of cardiovascular events, including heart failure, increases with pulse pressure.

Risk Enhancers in Hypertension

Hypertension progressing on to heart failure is usually associated with coronary disease, diabetes, left ventricular hypertrophy or valvular deformity, conditions also promoted by hypertension (Table 3). In hypertensive men going on to cardiac failure, 52%

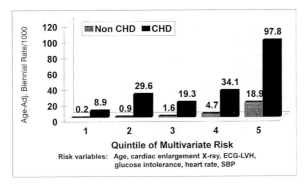

Fig. 1. Risk of cardiac failure by quintile of multivariate risk and CHD status. A 32-year follow-up – the Framingham study of men 35–94 years of Age

had myocardial infarctions; among hypertensive women it was 34%. Angina pectoris preceded hypertensive heart failure in 35% of either sex. Angina without accompanying infarction was less common (12%–21%). Conversely, coronary disease evolving on to heart failure is usually accompanied by hypertension.

Hypertension likely to progress on to heart failure is usually accompanied by left ventricular hypertrophy 20% of which manifested on the ECG and 60%–70% on the more sensitive echocardiogram. Heart failure risk increases progressively with left ventricular mass with no discernible value separating compensatory from pathological hypertrophy. Anatomical (roentgenographic or echocardiographic) and ECG manifestations of left ventricular hypertrophy each independently contribute to risk, and those subjects with both conditions have a substantially greater risk than those with either alone (Fig. 1).

In hypertensive persons a myocardial infarction increases the risk of progressing on to heart failure five- to sixfold (Table 4). Angina imposes a 1.4- to 7-fold increased risk in men and women, respectively. Diabetes and left ventricular hypertrophy each escalate the risk two- to threefold. Development of valvular heart disease increases the risk about twofold.

Epidemiologic investigation of heart failure has led to the identification of some useful indicators of deteriorating left ventricular function in the hypertensive patient such as a rapid resting heart rate [13], a low vital capacity [10], cardiac enlargement on a chest

Table 4. Predisposing conditions for heart failure in hypertension; Framingham study of subjects aged 40–89 years (from [12])

Condition	Sex	Age and risk factor-adjusted hazard ratio
Myocardial infarction	M	5.54
	F	5.99
Angina pectoris	M	1.35
	F	1.71
Diabetes	M	1.78
	F	3.57
Valvular heart disease	M	2.40
	F	1.96
Left ventricular hypertrophy	M	1.97
	F	2.80

The hazard ratio is adjusted for the other listed coexisting conditions. The multivariate hazard ratio for angina in men is not statistically significant.

film, and echocardiographic or ECG evidence of left ventricular hypertrophy. Hypertensive persons usually have higher resting heart rates, and the risk of hypertension evolving on to failure increases the higher the accompanying heart rate. A low or falling vital capacity is an ominous harbinger of heart failure in persons with hypertension, coronary disease or left ventricular hypertrophy.

Multivariate Risk Assessment

The epidemiologic identification of other independent predisposing contributors to the development of heart failure in persons with hypertension makes it possible to devise multivariable risk formulations to estimate their probability of developing heart failure conditional on the coexistent burden of other relevant risk factors [10]. A logistic function comprised of age, heart rate, vital capacity, systolic blood pressure, ECG evidence of left ventricular hypertrophy, cardiomegaly on chest X-ray, and the possibility of additional coronary disease or valvular heart disease makes it possible to identify one fifth of the hypertensive persons from which about 70% of the heart failure will arise [14]. Those in the

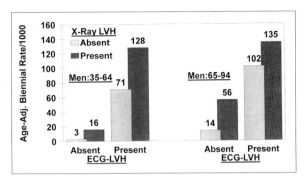

Fig. 2. Risk of cardiac failure by ECG and roentgenographic evidence of LVH. A 32-year follow-up of the Framingham study. (From [26])

upper quintile of multivariate risk, where the truly high risk of failure is concentrated, are good candidates for definitive diagnostic procedures to detect those subjects with left ventricular dysfunction who need vigorous preventive measures (Fig. 2). Quantifying the risk in this way helps to avoid overlooking the many high risk candidates for failure with multiple marginal predisposing abnormalities.

Preventive Implications

The epidemiologic data implicating hypertension as a prominent feature of heart failure satisfy a number of criteria for a causal connection, including the biological plausibility of the relationship, the strength of the association, persistence of the effect after adjustment for confounders, the temporal sequence of the relationship, the presence of a dose-response association, and the consistency of the finding in different samples [16, 17]. Major hypertension trials provide further support of causality by documenting that treatment of hypertension can reduce risk of cardiac failure [6, 18, 19]. A recent metaanalysis indicates that hypertension treatment can reduce heart failure in the elderly by as much as 47%, which is in close agreement with the population-attributable risk for development of hypertension-induced heart failure reported by the Framingham Study [12, 19]

Clinical trials have indicated that several medical interventions can improve survival in persons who have heart failure [6, 20–23], but the outlook is still poor [14, 16, 23, 24]. Mortality following the development of heart failure is unacceptably high. Median survival following the diagnosis of heart failure in Framingham study subjects was only 1.37 years in men and 2.48 years in women [15]. At 5 years of follow-up, 76% of men and 69% of women were dead. Despite improvement in survival with currently recommended therapy with ACE inhibitors and beta-blockers, once the failure is overtly manifested, the prognosis remains grave. Reduction of the incidence of heart failure and the high mortality it causes requires preventive strategies to detect and aggressively manage hypertension and the heart failure-promoting conditions that it induces in the presymptomatic stage. Therapy of the hypertensive candidate for heart failure now emphasizes seeking out and correcting presymptomatic left ventricular dysfunction and the maladaptive changes induced by deteriorating myocardial function.

Acknowledgements. Framingham Study research is supported by NIH/NHLBI Contract N01-HC-38038 and the Visiting Scientist Program, which is supported by Astra USA, Hoechst Marion Roussel and Servier Canada, Inc.

References

1. Graves EG, Billum BS (1996) 1994 summary: national hospital discharge survey: advance data. National Center for Health Statistics 278:1–12
2. National Heart, Lung and Blood Institute (1996) Data fact sheet: congestive heart failure in the USA: a new epidemic. NHLBI Information Center, Bethesda
3. National Heart, Lung and Blood Institute (1996) Morbidity and mortality chartbook on cardiovascular, lung and blood diseases. Bethesda
4. Kannel WB, Castelli WP, McNamara PM, McKee PA, Feinleib M (1972) Role of blood pressure in the development of congestive heart failure: the Framingham study. N Engl J Med 287:781–787
5. Ericksson H, Svardsudd K, Larsson B et al. (1989) Risk factors for heart failure in the general population: the study of men born in 1913. Eur Heart J 10:657–656

6. Pfeffer MA, Braunwald E, Moye LA et al. (1992) Effect of captopril on mortality and morbidity in patients with left ventricular dysfunction after myocardial infarction: results of the survical and ventricular enlargement trial. N Engl J Med 327:669–677
7. Teerlink JR, Goldhaber SZ, Pfeffer MA (1991) An overview of contemporary etiologies of congestive heart failure. Am Heart J 121:1852–1853
8. Kannel WB, Hjortland MC, Castelli WP (1974) Role of diabetes in congestive heart failure: the Framingham study. Am J Cardiol 34:29–34
9. Braunwald E (1992) Valvular heart disease. In: Braunwald E (ed) Heart disease. Saunders, Philadelphia, pp 1007–1077
10. Ho KK, Pinsky JL, Kannel WB, Levy D (1993) The epidemiology of heart failure: the Framingham study. J Am Coll Cardiol 22:6A–13A
11. Yusuf S, Thom T, Abbott RD (1989) Changes in hypertension treatment and in congestive heart failure mortality in the United States. Hypertension 13(Suppl I):174–179
12. Levy D, Larson MG, Vasan RS, Kannel WB, Ho KKL (1996) The progression from hypertension to congestive heart failure. JAMA 275:1557–1562
13. Gillman MW, Kannel WB, Belanger A, et al. (1993) Influence of heart rate on mortality among persons with hypertension: The Framingham study. Am Heart J 125:1148–1154
14. Kannel WB (1996) Need and prospects for prevention of heart failure. Eur J Clin Pharm 49:S 3–S 9
15. Ho KK, Anderson KM, Kannel WB, Grossman W, Levy D (1993) Survival after the onset of congestive heart failure in Framingham heart study subjects. Circulation 88:107–115
16. Hill BA (1965) The environment and disease: association or causation? Proc R Soc Med 58:295–300
17. Glenn JR (1993) A question of attribution. Lancet 342:530–532
18. Furberg CD, Yusuf S (1986) Effect of drug therapy on survival in chronic heart failure. Adv Cardiol 34:124–130
19. Cutler JA, Psaty BM, MacMahon S, Furberg CD (1995) Public health issues in hypertension control: what has been learned from clinical trials. In: Laragh JH, Brenner BH (eds) Hypertension: pathophysiology, diagnosis and management. Raven, New York, pp 253–270
20. Cohn JN, Johnson G, Ziesche S et al. (1991) A comparison of enalapril with hydralazine-isosorbide dinitrate in the treatment of chronic congestive heart failure. N Engl J Med 325:303–310
21. The SOLVD investigators (1991) Effect of enalapril on survical in patients with reduced left ventricular ejection fractions and congestive heart failure. N Engl J Med 325:393–302
22. Garg R, Yusuf S (1995) Overview of randomized trials of angiotensin-converting enzyme inhibitors on mortality and morbidity in patients with heart failure: collaborative group on ACE-inhibitor trials. JAMA 273:1450–1456
23. Packer M, Bristow MR, Cohen JN, Colucci WS, Fowler MB, Gilbert EM, Shusterman NH, for the Carvedilol Heart Failure Study Group (1996)

The effect of Carvedilol on morbidity and mortality in patients with chronic heart failure. N Engl J Med 334:1349–1355

24. Schocken DD, Arrieta MI, Leaverton PE, Ross EA (1992) Prevalence and mortality rate of congestive heart failure in the United States. J Am Coll Cardiol 20:301–306
25. Gillum RF (1987) Heart failure in the United States 1970–1985. Am Heart 113:1043–1045
26. Kannel WB, Ho K, Thom T (1994) The changing epidemiologic features of cardiac failure. Br Heart J 72:S 3–S 9

PART II

Hypertension

β-Blockers in the Treatment of Hypertension: Focus on Carvedilol

ANDERS HIMMELMANN

Introduction

The concept of α- and β-adrenoceptors was first described in 1948, and 10 years later the first β-blocking compound, dichlorisoprenaline, was discovered [1]. However, the idea of differing adrenergic receptors can be traced back to the beginning of the twentieth century, when excitatory and inhibitory effects of the administration of adrenaline or of sympathetic nerve stimulation were described [2]. The β-blocking compounds pronethalol and propranolol were initially used to treat patients with angina pectoris, cardiac arrhythmias, and pheochromocytoma, while the demonstration of their hypotensive effects was unexpected [1, 2]. Pronethalol was later withdrawn due to development of tumors in mice, whereas propranolol became the standard drug to assess all subsequent β-blocking agents.

Treatment of elevated arterial pressure with antihypertensive agents results in significant reductions in cardiovascular morbidity and mortality [3]. In a meta-analysis of 13 major intervention trials in hypertensive patients, a reduction in diastolic blood pressure of 5–6 mmHg was shown to reduce the incidence of stroke by 42% and that of coronary heart disease by 14%. In these trials β-blockers and diuretics were the drugs most often used. Moreover, the health outcomes associated with antihypertensive therapies used as first-line agents were evaluated in a recent meta-analysis [4]. Compared with placebo, β-blocker-based therapy was as effective as diuretic-based therapy in preventing stroke and congestive heart failure. In a randomized open trial in hypertensive men, the β-blocker metoprolol given as initial antihypertensive treatment reduced deaths from coronary heart disease and stroke, sudden death, and total mortality to a greater extent than the thiazide diuretics hydrochlorothiazide or bendroflumethiazide [5, 6]. Without doubt, the value of β-blockers as first-line antihypertensive agents is proven [3, 4, 7].

Pharmacology

Pharmacodynamics

β-Blockers are classified into nonselective drugs which block both β-1 and β-2 adrenergic receptors, e.g., propranolol and alprenolol, and β-1 selective, e.g., atenolol and metoprolol. Some β-blockers also possess ancillary properties such as intrinsic sympathomimetic activity (pindolol), α-adrenoceptor blocking activity (labetalol), or class III antiarrhythmic effect (sotalol).

Carvedilol is a multiple-action compound with a nonselective β-blocking effect combined with a vasodilating action based on α-adrenoceptor blockade [8]. In addition, carvedilol exerts a number of well documented ancillary effects such as being a scavenger of free radicals and it also has an antiproliferative action on smooth muscle cells. This combination of effects opens up a number of interesting clinical perspectives.

Pharmacokinetics

β-Blockers are rapidly absorbed, but undergo an extensive and variable first-pass metabolism in the liver resulting in differences in bioavailability. They also differ with regard to lipophilicity. Lipid-soluble drugs are metabolized in the liver, while water-soluble compounds are excreted by the kidney.

Carvedilol is also rapidly absorbed and the compound undergoes extensive first-pass hepatic metabolism which results in a bioavailability of 25% [9]. It is highly lipophilic and its metabolism is primarily hepatic. Since less than 2% of a dose is excreted unchanged in the urine, dosage adjustment in patients with renal impairment is not required.

Mode of Action

The mechanism by which β-blockers lower blood pressure is not clear, and the mechanism may not be the same in all patients [1, 2, 10]. Several theories have been advanced to explain the hypotensive effect(s) of β-blockers. These include the reduction in cardiac output and, during chronic treatment, long-term reduction in peripheral resistance, direct action on the central nervous system, presynaptic blocking of adrenergic neurones, suppression of renin release, stimulation of vasodilator prostaglandins, resetting of arterial baroreceptors, an effect on plasma volume, and an increase in the levels of the atrial natriuretic peptide.

Hemodynamic Effects

Invasive hemodynamic studies following acute administration of carvedilol have shown that blood pressure falls promptly due to a numeric, but statistically insignificant, reduction of cardiac output while total peripheral resistance remains unchanged [11]. All these effects are in contrast to the acute effects of a pure β-blocker such as propranolol given intravenously to hypertensive patients [10]. This does not lower blood pressure acutely, in spite of causing a marked drop in cardiac output, which is explained by an equally great increase in total peripheral resistance [11]. In a double-blind comparison with propranolol in patients with essential hypertension, carvedilol did not reduce forearm blood flow, in contrast to propranolol [12].

In a short-term randomized hemodynamic comparison between carvedilol and metoprolol it was confirmed that cardiac output did not change with carvedilol even after 4 weeks of treatment, whereas a significant reduction was seen in the metoprolol-treated patients [13]. An improvement of left ventricular diastolic function has also been described with carvedilol treatment both in hypertensives and in patients with ischemic heart disease [14].

The long-term hemodynamic effects of carvedilol when used for the treatment of hypertension are: a significant reduction in systolic and diastolic blood pressure, a reduction in total peripheral

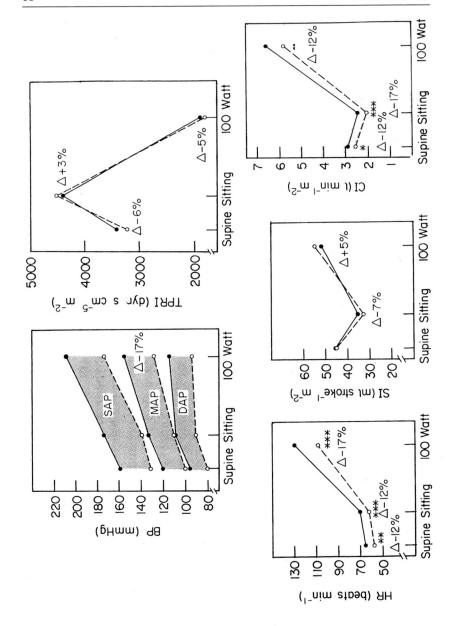

resistance, a slight fall in heart rate, and little or no change in cardiac output (Fig. 1) [15].

Clinical Effects

Blood Pressure Reduction

β-Blockers effectively lower an elevated blood pressure [1, 2, 10]. The reduction in blood pressure with *β*-blockade is usually proportional to the initial blood pressure level [2]. They usually have a pronounced effect within the first few days, and by 2–3 weeks almost all of the effect has been achieved.

Carvedilol has in comparative trials shown to be of equivalent efficacy to other *β*-blockers, thiazide diuretics, angiotensin-converting enzyme (ACE) inhibitors, and calcium antagonists [9, 16]. Its efficacy has also been demonstrated in combination therapy with either a thiazide diuretic or a calcium antagonist [9].

Effects on Other Risk Factors

Glucose and Lipid Metabolism

β-Blockers tend to worsen insulin resistance and deteriorate lipoprotein metabolism, while angiotensin-converting enzyme inhibitors and calcium antagonists are neutral, and *α*-blockers improve these factors [17]. In fact, these unbeneficial effects of *β*-blockers and diuretics, as compared to other classes of antihypertensive

Fig. 1. Changes in hemodynamic variables during chronic treatment with carvedilol supine, sitting, and during 100-W exercise. *SAP* systolic arterial pressure; *MAP*, mean arterial pressure; *DAP*, diastolic arterial pressure; *BP*, blood pressure; *TPRI*, total peripheral resistance index; *HR*, heart rate; *SI*, stroke index; *CI*, cardiac index. *Filled circles* before treatment and *open circles* on carvedilol. D shows major changes. *$p<0.05$, **$p<0.01$, ***$p<0.001$. All changes in blood pressure are highly significant, but significance asterisks are not shown in the figure. (From [15])

drugs, may explain the poor effect on risk of coronary heart disease in intervention trials [3].

Carvedilol does not unfavorably affect glucose and lipid metabolism in either nondiabetic or diabetic patients with hypertension [18, 19]. In a multicenter double-blind trial, 72 nondiabetic hypertensive patients were randomly assigned to treatment with either carvedilol or metoprolol [18]. An isoglycemic, hyperinsulinemic glucose clamp was conducted at baseline and after 12 weeks of treatment. After metoprolol treatment, insulin sensitivity decreased significantly by about 14%, whereas it increased after carvedilol treatment. There was also a decrease in high-density lipoprotein and an increase in triglyceride level in patients in the metoprolol-treated group, whereas these variables remained unchanged in patients in the carvedilol-treated group.

A randomized, double-blind, 24-week trial was conducted in 45 diabetic patients with hypertension to compare the metabolic effects of carvedilol with those of atenolol [19]. Fasting plasma glucose and insulin levels decreased with carvedilol and increased with atenolol. Carvedilol also more favorably affected lipid metabolism, i.e., there was a decrease in triglyceride level and increase in high-density lipoprotein cholesterol level.

Left Ventricular Hypertrophy

Left ventricular hypertrophy has been recognized as a very potent risk indicator of cardiovascular morbidity [20]. Preventive strategies directed toward earlier and more aggressive blood pressure control may slow the progression from hypertension to heart failure [21]. Numerous studies, e.g., summarized in a meta-analysis, have shown that β-blockers reduce left ventricular mass [22]. Several studies with carvedilol have shown that this compound rapidly and substantially reduces left ventricular mass [23, 24, 25]. The effects of carvedilol on left ventricular function and mass were studied in hypertensive patients with diastolic filling abnormalities. Treatment produced significant decreases in left ventricular mass and left ventricular mass index [23]. There were coincident improvements in diastolic left ventricular function. In another study, 3 months of treatment with carvedilol in hypertensive patients caused a reduction in left ventricular mass in individual patients and, after 6 months, a significant reduction in ventricular wall thickness [24]. In a controlled study, in patients with mild to moderate hypertension and left ventricular hypertrophy, carvedilol produced significant reductions in interventricular septum thickness and posterior wall thickness [25].

Tolerability and Safety

Most adverse reactions associated with *β*-blockade are predictable from the pharmacodynamic features of the drugs, and are obviously mediated by the adrenoceptor antagonism, whereas some serious adverse reactions which have been associated with certain *β*-blockers, such as the oculomucocutaneous syndrome with practolol and liver necrosis with dilevalol, are probably not related to the *β*-blockade *per se* [2]. Common *β*-blocker-induced side effects include fatigue and lethargy, while bronchoconstriction, gastrointestinal annoyance, sexual dysfunction, and sleep disturbance occur less commonly, and heart failure and second- or third-degree heart block are very rare.

In comparison with other *β*-blockers, and diuretics, calcium antagonists, and angiotensin-converting enzyme inhibitors, and in combination therapy, carvedilol has generally been well tolerated, with few side effects. In an 8-week double-blind study in 325 patients with hypertension, in which 25 mg carvedilol once daily was compared to 50 mg atenolol, adverse experiences were reported by 22% of patients who received carvedilol and by 21% of patients who were given atenolol [26]. The most common adverse experiences were headache, dizziness, and somnolence in the carvedilol group and dizziness and fatigue in the atenolol group.

The safety of carvedilol has been summarized from reports of 908 patients treated with carvedilol in clinical trials [27]. Headache was the most common adverse reaction, occurring in 5.7% of the patients, while dizziness was reported in 4.8%, tiredness in 2.2%, orthostatic reactions in 1.6%, weakness in 1.5%, nausea in 1.3%, and malaise in 0.9%. Serious adverse events occurring during clinical trials with carvedilol have been few, but include three episodes of reversible thrombocytopenia which were not clearly caused by the drug, two episodes of urticaria, one complete heart block, and one myocardial infarction possibly related to drug treatment [28].

A postmarketing surveillance study of 2226 patients treated with carvedilol for 12 weeks has been presented [29]. Adverse events caused the withdrawal of therapy in 164 patients, while 65 withdrew because of lack of efficacy and 20 withdrew for other reasons. The most common adverse events causing discontinuation of treatment were vertigo in 1.7%, headache in 1.4%, and in 0.5% bronchospasm, fatigue, and skin reactions, respectively.

The long-term efficacy and safety of carvedilol were investigated, over a period of 1 year, in an open clinical study of 154 patients with essential hypertension [30]. Eight patients dropped out because they were nonresponders, and another eight because of adverse events. Most of the reported side effects were characteristic of β-blockers, i.e., lethargy, headache, and bradycardia.

Although headache was among the most frequently reported side effects in clinical trials [27], in the postmarketing surveillance study [29] and in long-term treatment [30] it is worth noting that the incidence of headache decreased significantly with carvedilol treatment as compared to the placebo period when symptoms were evaluated with the "Göteborg Quality of Life Assessment" [31].

Quality of Life

Studies of quality of life in patients treated with β-blockers have not been consistent [2]. In one study, propranolol treatment caused deterioration of general wellbeing and more complaints of sexual dysfunction, as compared to patients who received an ACE inhibitor [32]. Quality of life in hypertensive patients treated with either carvedilol or the ACE inhibitor enalapril was studied by Östergren et al. [31]. In a 5-month maintenance period, after the

⟶

Fig. 2. Representation of symptom profiles during treatment with carvedilol and enalapril. *Thin lines* indicate frequency (%) of each symptom during placebo treatment and *thick lines* frequency during active treatment. (From [31])

Treatment Carvedilol, Symptoms profile (%)

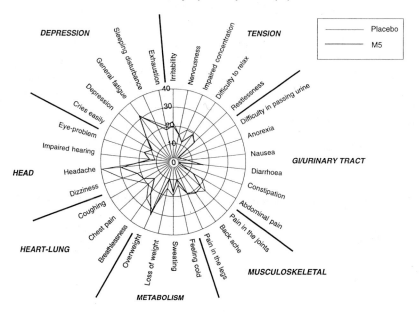

Treatment Enalapril, Symptoms profile (%)

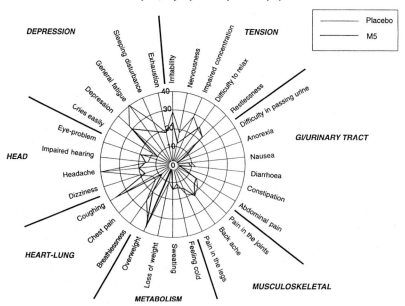

patients had reached the goal blood pressure 90 mmHg, quality of life was evaluated using the "Göteborg Quality of Life Assessment" [31]. For most items, no significant differences were found between the treatments (Fig. 2). Cough was a more common complaint in the enalapril group, while there were no differences between the treatments with regard to typical β-blocker-related symptoms, e.g., quality of sleep, occurrence of nightmares, sexual interest and ability, cold hands or feet, and perceived degree of energy.

Summary

In summary, the therapeutic efficacy of carvedilol has been amply documented in hypertension. It lowers elevated blood pressure effectively, and affects other cardiovascular risk factors in a neutral or positive manner. In addition, in patients with congestive heart failure and ischemic heart disease carvedilol provides additional benefit in terms of reduced mortality and morbidity [33, 34].

References

1. Bolli P, Fernandez PG, Bühler FR(1990) Beta-blockers in the treatment of hypertension. In: Laragh JH, Brenner BM (eds) Hypertension, diagnosis, and management. Raven Press, New York, pp 2181–2208
2. Prichard BNC, Cruickshank JM (1995) Beta blockade in hypertension: past, present, and future. In: Laragh JH, Brenner BM (eds) Hypertension, diagnosis, and management, 2nd edn. Raven Press, New York, pp 2827–2859
3. Collins R, Peto R, MacMahon S, Hebert P, Fiebach NH, Eberlein KA, Godwin J, Qizilbash N, Taylor JO, Hennekens CH (1990) Blood pressure, stroke, and coronary heart disease. Part 2, Short-term reductions in blood pressure: overview of randomised drug trials in their epidemiological context. Lancet 335:827–838
4. Psaty BM, Smith NL, Siscovick DS, Koepsell TD, Weiss NS, Heckbert SR, Lemaitre RN, Wagner EH, Furberg CD (1997) Health outcomes associated with antihypertensive therapies used as first-line agents. A systematic review and meta-analysis. JAMA 277:739–745
5. Wikstrand J, Warnold I, Olsson G, Tuomilehto J, Elmfeldt D, Berglund G (1988) Primary prevention with metoprolol in patients with hypertension. Mortality results from the MAPHY study. JAMA 259:1976–1982

6. Olsson G, Tuomilehto J, Berglund G, et al. (1991) Primary prevention of sudden cardiovascular death in hypertensive patients: mortality results from the MAPHY study. Am J Hypertens 4:151–158
7. Zanchetti A, Chalmers JP, Arakawa K, Gyarfas I, Hamet P, Hansson L, Julius S, MacMahon S, Mancia G, Ménard J, Omae T, Reid J, Safar M (1993) The 1993 guidelines for the management of mild hypertension: memorandum from a WHO/ISH meeting. Blood Pressure 2:86–100
8. Ruffolo RR Jr, Gellai M, Hieble JP, Willette RN, Nichols AJ (1990) The pharmacology of carvedilol. Eur J Clin Pharmacol 38(Suppl 10):S82–S88
9. McTavish D, Campoli-Richards D, Sorkin EM (1993) Carvedilol. A review of its pharmacodynamic and pharmacokinetic properties, and therapeutic efficacy. Drugs 45:232–258
10. Hansson L (1996) *β*-adrenoreceptor blockers in hypertension. In: Messerli FH (ed) Cardiovascular drug therapy, 2nd edn. WB Saunders, Philadelphia, pp 474–483
11. Eggertsen R, Andren L, Sivertsson R, Hansson L (1984) Acute haemodynamic effects of carvedilol (BM 14190), a new combined beta-adrenoceptor blocker and precapillary vasodilating agent, in hypertensive patients. Eur J Clin Pharmacol 27:19–22
12. Eggertsen R, Sivertsson R, Andrén L, Hansson L (1984) Haemodynamic effects of carvedilol, a new beta-adrenoceptor blocker and precapillary vasodilator in essential hypertension. J Hypertens 2:529–534
13. Weber K, Bohemeke T, van der Does R, Taylor SH (1996) Comparison of the hemodynamic effects of metoprolol and carvedilol in hypertensive patients. Cardiovasc Drug Ther 10:113–117
14. Lahiri A, Rodrigues EA, Heber ME, van der Does R, Raftery EB (1988) Effects of carvedilol on left ventricular function in hypertension and ischemic heart disease. Drugs 36(Suppl 2):141–144
15. Lund-Johansen P, Omvik P (1992) Chronic haemodynamic effects of carvedilol in essential hypertension at rest and during exercise. Eur Heart J 13:281–286
16. Dunn CJ, Lea AP, Wagstaff AJ (1997) Carvedilol. A reappraisal of its pharmacological properties and therapeutic use in cardiovascular disorders. Drugs 54:161–185
17. Lithell HOL (1991) Effect of antihypertensive drugs on insulin, glucose and lipid metabolism. Diabetes Care 14:203–209
18. Jacob S, Rett K, Wicklmayr M, Agrawal B, Augustin HJ, Dietze GJ (1996) Differential effect of chronic treatment with two beta-blocking agents on insulin sensitivity: the carvedilol–metoprolol study. J Hypertens 14:489–494
19. Giugliano D, Acampora R, Marfella R, De RN, Ziccardi P, Ragone R, De Angelis L, D'Onofrio F (1997) Metabolic and cardiovascular effects of carvedilol and atenolol in non-insulin-dependent diabetes mellitus and hypertension. A randomized, controlled trial. Ann Intern Med 126:955–959

20. Levy D, Garrison RJ, Savage DD, Kannel WB, Castelli WP (1990) Prognostic implications of echocardiographically determined left ventricular mass in the Framingham Heart Study. N Engl J Med 322:1561–1566

21. Levy D, Larsson MG, Vasan RS, Kannel WB, Ho KKL (1996) The progression from hypertension to congestive heart failure. JAMA 275:1557–1562

22. Schmieder RE, Martus P, Klingbeil A (1996) Reversal of left ventricular hypertrophy in essential hypertension. A meta-analysis of randomized double-blind studies. JAMA 275:1507–1513

23. Why HJ, Richardson PJ (1992) Effect of carvedilol on left ventricular function and mass in hypertension. J Cardiovasc Pharmacol 19(Suppl 1): S50–S54

24. Eichstaedt H, Schroeder RJ, Auffermann W, Richter W (1992) Regression of left ventricular hypertrophy. J Cardiovasc Pharmacol 19(Suppl 1):S55–S61

25. Schroeder R-J, Cordes M, Danne O, Eichstädt HW (1994) Left ventricular hypertrophy regression and cardiac function under antihypertensive therapy – a comparison of a vasodilating beta adrenoceptor blocker and an ACE-inhibitor. Perfusion 7:210–218

26. Ruilope LM (1994) Comparison of a new vasodilating beta-blocker, carvedilol, with atenolol in the treatment of mild to moderate essential hypertension. Am J Hypertens 7:129–136

27. Abshagen U (1987) A new molecule with vasodilating and beta-adrenoceptor blocking properties. J Cardiovasc Pharmacol 10(Suppl 11):S23–S32

28. Carlsson WD, Gilbert EM (1996) Carvedilol. In: Messerli FH (ed) Cardiovascular drug therapy, 2nd edn. WB Saunders, Philadelphia, pp 583–599

29. Cauchie P, Vanden Abeele C, Biemans M, Mattelaer P (1992) A prospective postmarketing surveillance study of carvedilol in the management of hypertension in general practice. J Hypertens 10:191

30. Schnurr E, Widmann L, Glocke M (1987) Efficacy and safety of carvedilol in the treatment of hypertension. J Cardiovasc Pharmacol 10(Suppl 11):S101–S107

31. Östergren J, Storstein L, Karlberg BE, Tibblin G (1996) Quality of life in hypertensive patients treated with either carvedilol or enalapril. Blood Pressure 5:41–49

32. Croog SH, Levine S, Testa MA, Brown B, Bulpit CJ, Jenkins CD, Klerman GL, Williams GH (1986) The effects of antihypertensive therapy on the quality of life. N Engl J Med 314:1657–1664

33. Packer M, Bristow MR, Cohn JN, Colucci WS, Fowler MB, Gilbert EM, Shusterman NH, for the US Carvedilol Heart Failure Study (1996) The effect of carvedilol on morbidity and mortality in patients with chronic heart failure. N Engl J Med 334:1349–1355

34. Basu S, Senior R, Raval U, van der Does R, Bruchner T, Lahiri A (1997) Beneficial effects of intravenous and oral carvedilol treatment in acute myocardial infarction. A placebo-controlled, randomized trial. Circulation 96:183–191

Ergometry in the Assessment of Arterial Hypertension and Antihypertensive Therapy

I.-W. FRANZ

Introduction

Evaluation of high blood pressure could be greatly facilitated by a standardized test procedure enabling comparable and reproducible blood pressure determination. Furthermore a standardized method for monitoring sympathetic activity could be useful in more accurately assessing the occurrence and magnitude of inordinate stress responses. One way of meeting these requirements is through standardized ergometric testing [9, 10, 12].

Methods of Test Performance

We recommend a range of 50–100 W with increments of 10 W/min or 25 W/min because this range corresponds well with ordinary levels of exertion. Since even exercise of such an intensity can elicit marked blood pressure elevations [10, 16, 32], the vascular risk of arterial hypertension is accurately characterized by this range [9, 10].

Blood pressure readings were taken at 1-min intervals during the last 20 s of each minute, during ergometry as well as for 5 min during the recovery period. There is a general agreement that indirect measurements yield systolic blood pressure readings insignificantly different from direct intravascular measurements [2, 31, 38].

By contrast, Matthes et al. [31] and Rost [38] reported that direct and indirect measurements of diastolic pressure correlate well only for very mild ergometric workloads.

One criterion for the significance of blood pressure control during ergometry is the reproducibility of results. Lassvik [27] calculated a coefficient of variation of maximum blood pressure response of 3%+2% (mean+SD, within 1 day) and of 5%+4% (mean+SD, day-to-day). Good reproducibility was also reported by others [6, 13, 18]. In untreated patients with borderline and mild hypertension, blood pressure measurements repeated three times during ergometric testing agreed well with a mean of 203/116 mmHg at 8 a.m., 200/114 mmHg at 10 a.m. and 203/113 mmHg at 4 p.m., although resting blood pressures differed significantly at times [13].

Normal Values of Blood Pressure

A total of 323 normotensive men and women (20 to 50 years of age) of varying occupations was recruited from the staffs of three major Berlin companies in order to obtain the normal blood pressure response during and after ergometry (Fig. 1) [10, 14]. The maximum normal values discussed here for blood pressure during and after ergometry refer to the mean values plus one standard deviation.

Between the ages of 20 and 50 years the criteria for a hypertensive response during exercise were blood pressure values of more than 200/100 mmHg (mean+1 SD of the normotensives) at a workload of 100 W and corresponding heart rates of 126±13 beats/min [14]. In the recovery phase, blood pressure was considered as being hypertensive if a value of 140/90 mmHg was exceeded during the fifth minute. At least three of these parameters had to apply for blood pressure response to be classified as hypertensive.

For 51- to 70-year-old men and women it is necessary to employ higher blood pressure limits during and after exercise [10, 16]. For this group a blood pressure of 200/105 mmHg is considered to be the maximum normal value for a 70-W workload, and 215/105 mmHg maximum normal value for 100 W. After the fifth minute of recovery, blood pressure should not exceed 150/90 mmHg.

These values are in good agreement with the data of Gleichmann [17] and Samek et al. [39] as well as other investigators [1, 23, 29]. Heck et al. [22] reported markedly lower blood pressures at 100 W with a risk of false-positive results.

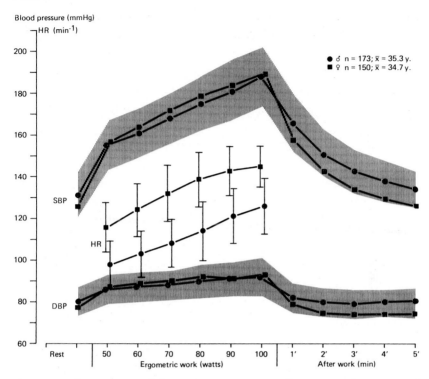

Blood pressure (mmHg)

HR (min⁻¹)

♂ n = 173; x̄ = 35.3 y.
♀ n = 150; x̄ = 34.7 y.

SBP

HR

DBP

Rest   50   60   70   80   90   100   1'   2'   3'   4'   5'
          Ergometric work (watts)   After work (min)

Fig. 1. Blood pressure and heart rate responses of normotensive men and women 20 to 50 years of age

Ergometry in the Predicition of Hypertension in Patients with Normal Resting Blood Pressure

There are serveral studies [5, 7, 21, 33, 41, 42], showing that blood pressure reactivity to exercise is an indication of future resting blood pressure. In a cohort of 1184 men and 1385 women free of cardiovascular disease and hypertension who were studied between 1979 and 1983 in the Framingham offspring study [21], systolic blood pressure response during exercise predicted the 4-year incidence of hypertension in men.

Ergometry in the Assessment of Arterial Hypertension Classification into Normal and High Blood pressure

The potential application of ergometry as a diagnostic tool will be shown from the data of one of our studies [10, 12, 16] comprising 475 men: 173 normotensives (mean age 35.3±7.3 years), 98 borderline hypertensives (mean age 36.7±9.6 years), 204 hypertensives (mean age 38.5±7.2 years) aged 20 to 50 years.

Normotensive Patients. In normotensive patients, systolic blood pressure continuously increased with each increment from 155±12 mmHg at 50 W to 188±14 mmHg at 100 W (Fig. 2).

Diastolic blood pressure increased only slightly during exercise from 86±7 mmHg at 50 W to 92±9 mmHg at 100 W. After exercise, systolic blood pressure (138±10 mmHg) returned to the normotensive range within 4 min, whereas diastolic blood pressure returned to normal within the first minute of the recovery period (82±7 mmHg).

Hypertensive Patients. The patients suffering from mild hypertension in group 1A (<170/<105 mmHg, <50 years) showed significantly higher systolic blood pressure (p <0.001) and in particular higher diastolic (p <0.001) blood pressure than the normotensives during and after exercise. Figure 2 clearly demonstrates that groups of hypertensive patients with higher blood pressure values at rest [group 1B (>170/>105 mmHg, <50 years) compared with group 1A] on average also showed higher systolic ($p<0.001$) and diastolic ($p<0.001$) blood pressures during and after exercise.

Borderline Hypertensive Patients. Using the normal maximum values for blood pressure in men between the ages of 20 and 50 years (200/100 mmHg compared with a mean+1 SD for normotensives) at a workload of 100 W (corresponding heart rates of 126+13 beats/min) and a value of 140/90 mmHg in the fifth minute of the recovery period, the ergometric procedure revealed that 50% of the hypertensives who were borderline at rest could be classified as positive according to the test (Fig. 2). Their blood pressure response did not significantly differ during exercise (216/113 mmHg

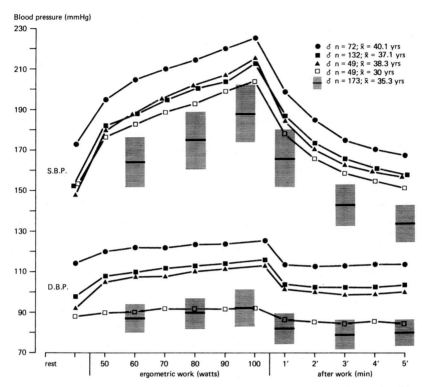

Fig. 2. Systolic (*S.B.P.*) and diastolic (*D.B.P.*) blood pressures (*mean values*) at rest and during and after exercise in patients with mild (*filled squares*, group 1A) and stable (*circles*, group 1B) hypertension an in borderline hypertensives who reacted negatively (*empty squares*) or positively (*triangles*) to the ergometric test. *Columns* indicate the normotensive range (mean±SD) of blood pressure during and after ergometry

at 100 W) or after ergometric exercise from that of age-matched patients with established hypertension (group 1A) whose blood pressure increased to 213/116 mmHg at 100 W. However, systolic and diastolic blood pressures were significantly higher ($p < 0.001$) than those of normotensives under all conditions. Thus, the subjects were classified as hypertensives.

In contrast, in the 50% of subjects who reacted negatively to the ergometric test, the systolic blood pressure response of 204 mmHg at 100 W during exercise was significantly ($p < 0.05$ to $p < 0.001$) lower than that of subjects showing a positive reaction and the hypertensives of group 1A. The pattern of the diastolic blood pressure is particularly worth noting. Patients showing a negative response revealed exactly the same diastolic blood pressure value of 92 mmHg at 100 W as the normotensives. In the fifth minute of the recovery period, the diastolic blood pressure of 85 mmHg in the negative patients was significantly lower (p <0.05) than the value of 88 mmHg before exercise. In contrast, diastolic blood pressure values of the ergometrically positive borderline hypertensives and the hypertensives (group 1A) with 97 mmHg and 104 mmHg, respectively, were significantly higher than 92 mmHg (p <0.01) and 98 mmHg (p <0.01), respectively, before exercise. Thus, ergometry enables investigators to disclose white-coat hypertensives as ergometric-negative during exercise. Follow-up examinations after 3.8 years showed that 97% of the ergometric-positive borderline hypertensives had developed chronic hypertension. Thus, early diagnosis of arterial hypertension was achieved by ergometry years before its manifestation. Conversely, 68% of patients with ergometric-negative borderline hypertension continued to demonstrate normotensive blood pressure during the follow-up period.

As also shown in other studies [1, 3, 9, 10, 23, 28, 30, 32, 40], systolic blood pressure in this study increased in relation to workload in both normotensives and hypertensives. However, the response of diastolic blood pressure to ergometric exercise is quite different among hyertensive and normotensive subjects [1, 3, 9, 10, 28, 32, 39]. Due to metabolic vasodilation during exercise, total peripheral resistance in normotensives decreases sharply, whereas the diastolic blood pressure remains unchanged or shows only a slight increase during submaximal ergometric exercise. However, hypertensive patients are characterized by a rise in diastolic blood pressure both during and after exercise.

This is further indicated by invasive hemodynamic exercise studies performed by Lund-Johansen [30] in 17- to 29-year-old patients with mild hypertension. Over a 10-year period these patients experienced only a slight change in their resting hemodynamics, while their total peripheral resistance and diastolic blood pressure during ergometry underwent a marked increase.

This hemodynamic pattern can be explained by the inability of hypertensive patients to reduce peripheral resistance during exercise to the same extent as normotensive subjects.

Impaired endothelium function during the early stage and subsequent reduced lumen-to-wall thickness could be responsible for increased resistance during exercise.

Taking into account the fact that stable arterial hypertension is characterized by increased peripheral resistance at rest and during exercise [30, 40], the differing behavior of diastolic blood pressure in normotensives and hypertensives during and after exercise is clinically significant in differentiating between normal and elevated blood pressures. This was also clearly demonstrated by the fact that neither the 173 normotensives nor the 204 hypertensives revealed a diastolic blood pressure response at 100 W that was higher or lower than 100 mmHg, respectively [9, 11]. Furthermore, in the fifth minute of the recovery phase none of the normotensives or hypertensives showed a diastolic blood pressure above or below the limit of 90 mmHg, respectively. Even in the young group (1A) with mild hypertension 74,2% revealed a diastolic blood pressure of more than 100 mmHg, whereas 15.2% had values between 95 mmHg and 99 mmHg and 10.6% between 90 mmHg and 94 mmHg.

The characteristic pattern of diastolic blood pressure during and after exercise in hypertensive patients has been confirmed by several other authors using direct and indirect methods [1, 3, 9, 10, 23, 24, 28, 32].

Prognosis of Cardiovascular Complications

Measurement of blood pressure at rest obviously involves uncertainty as to the presence of pathologically elevated blood pressure in response to daily physical and mental stress [10, 16], which may well be a decisive factor in determining the risk of hypertension [18, 26].

There is good evidence from various studies [18, 20, 34, 36, 37] that there is a significant correlation between systolic blood pressure during exercise and left-ventricular mass as assessed by echocardiography.

Moreover, pathological increases in exercise blood pressures suggest a considerable increase in myocardial oxygen consumption [10, 16] with an enhanced risk for myocardial ischemia in patients with CAD [35] and coronary microangiopathy [11, 15, 16].

In a long-term study Kjeldsen et al. [26] have clearly demonstrated that an abnormal response of systolic blood pressure during exercise predicts the development of typical organ damage.
The outcome of 1999 apparently healthy men aged 40–59 years
and examined from 1972 to 1975 was ascertained after 16 years to
determine if systolic blood pressure measured during a bicycle
ergometer exercise thest (workload of 100 W) predicted morbidity
and mortality from myocardial infarction beyond that of casual
blood pressure measured after 5 min of supine rest. During a total
follow-up of 31 984 patient years, 235 subjects had myocardial infarction, 143 cases of which were nonfatal and 92 fatal. Among the
520 men with casual systolic blood pressure >140 mmHg, there
were 304 who increased their systolic blood presure to >200
mmHg during 6 min of the initial exercise workload of 100 W.
These men ($n = 304$) had an excessive risk for myocardial infarction (18.8% vs 9.5% among the 1294 men with casual blood pressure <140 mmHg and exercise blood pressure <200 mmHg, p
<0.001). As many as 58% (33/57) of those men with myocardial
infarction in this group died, as opposed to 33% (range 26%–
35%) in all other groups ($p = 0.0011$), including those men with
casual blood pressure >140 mmHg and exercise blood pressure
<200 mmHg ($n=216$). In the group with increased systolic exer-
cise blood pressure and casual reading >140 mmHg, the cardiovascular mortality rate was 16.1%, as opposed to 5.6% in those
men with normal casual and exercise blood pressures.

Antihypertensive Drugs and Ergometry

The current goal of antihypertensive treatment is to normalize
resting blood pressure. However, this approach neglects basic
pathophysiological processes involved in arterial hypertension.
During physical exertion or emotional stress, the strain on the
heart and the load imposed on the vascular bed by a stress-linked
blood pressure rise are substantially increased relative to the resting state. It is therefore desirable to protect the cardiovascular system from the elevated blood pressure elicited by physical and
emotional stress. Antihypertensive drugs must not only normalize
the resting blood pressure but also lower blood pressure ade-

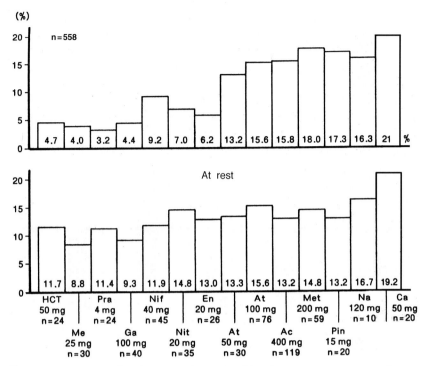

Fig. 3. Percentage of reduction of systolic blood pressure at rest and at a workload of 100 W after a 4-week treatment period with different kinds of hypertensive drugs in 538 previously untreated hypertensives. *HCT*, hydrochlorothiazide; *Me*, mefruside; *Pra*, prazosin; *Ga*, gallopamil; *Nif* nifedipine; *Nit*, nitrendipine; *En*, nalapril; *At*, atenolol; *Ac*,acebutolol; *Met*,metroprolol; *Pi*, pindolol; *Na*,nadolol; *Ca*, carvedilol

quately in stressful situations. This requirement is by no means met by all hypertensive drugs that are effective at rest [8, 10, 12, 16].

Figure 3 shows the effects of various antihypertensive drugs on blood pressure at rest and during exercise at a work rate of 100 W. Despite an identical systolic blood pressure reduction under testing conditions, the effect during exercise was significantly different.

β-blocking agents lower systolic blood pressure most effectively during dynamic exercise. Calcium antagonists also lower systolic blood pressure significantly during exercise, but to a lesser extent

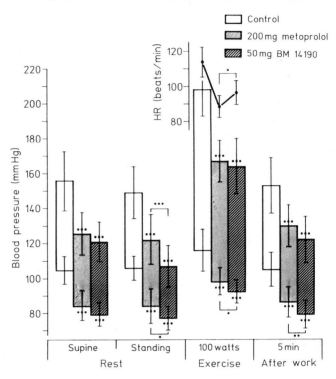

Fig. 4. Blood pressure and heart rate under resting, exercise and post-exercise conditions during control period and after 4 weeks of treatment with metoprolol and carvedilol in hypertensives ($n=20$, mean±SD) *p <0.05; ***p <0.001

that β-blockers. Diuretics, ACE inhibitors and prazosin have only a minor effect on systolic blood pressure elevation during exercise. The pharmacological profile of carvedilol includes both β-adrenoceptor blockade and vasodilation, the latter primarily a result of α-1-adrenoceptor blockade. Since arterial hypertension is considered to be a disease associated mainly with an increase in total peripheral resistance, carvedilol promises to be an interesting substance from the pathophysiological as well as clinical standpoint.

In a randomized, double-blind crossover study involving two 4-week periods of treatment with 50 mg carvedilol per day and 200 mg metoprolol per day, respectively we could show that carvedilol is at least as effective as metoprolol in reducing systolic blood pressure and much more effective in reducing diastolic blood pressure at rest and during exercise [16]. Heart rate was reduced significantly less by carvedilol than by metoprolol. This underlines the major contribution of vasodilation to the antihypertensive effect of carvedilol (Fig. 4). Regarding similar or even greater reduction of (diastolic) blood pressure during exercise, the smaller reduction of heart rate in patients receiving carvedilol is similar to physiological regulation. In spite of this, the reduction of the rate-pressure product (HR × SBP) is sufficient to imply much lower myocardial oxygen requirement, which has proven beneficial in the treatment of angina pectoris.

A subgroup analysis revealed that carvedilol was also effective in reducing blood pressure in those patients whose diastolic blood pressure was not sufficiently controlled by metoprolol (90 mmHg or more under supine resting conditions). These eight patients had an untreated blood pressure of 163±4/107±2 mmHg, a blood pressure of 136±3/93±2 mmHg with metoprolol, and a blood pressure of 123±3/80±2 mmHg with carvedilol (p <0.05). In the 12 other patients there was no significant difference in blood pressure reduction under supine resting conditions as brought about by the two β-blocking agents.

References

1. Anschelewitsch JV (1993) Blutdruckverhalten normotensiver und hypertensiver Personen während Ergometrie. In: Franz I-W (ed) Belastungsblutdruck bei Hochdruckkranken. Springer, Berlin Heidelberg New York, pp 579–583
2. Anschütz F (1970) Über die Zuverlässigkeit der auskultatorisch ermittelten Blutdruckwerte unter körperlicher Belastung. Fortschr Med 88:1391–1396
3. Bachour G, Bender F, Wessel F (1997) Telemetrische Überprüfung der normalen und gestörten arteriellen Blutdruckregulation unter Belastung. Med Welt 28:113–117
4. Bevegard S, Holmgren A, Jonsson B (1960) The effect of body position on the circulation at rest and during exercise with special reference to the influence on the stroke volume. Acta Physiol Scand 49:279–285
5. Briedigkeit W (1993) Untersuchungen zur Blutdruckentwicklung bei Kindern, Jugendlichen und jungen Erwachsenen unter besonderer Berück-

sichtigung des Belastungsblutdruckes. In: Franz I–W (ed) Belastungsblut-druck bei Hochdruckkranken. Springer, Berlin Heidelberg New York, pp 595–1000

6. Caen JL, Faurie A, Debru JL, Can G, Maillion JM (1978) Reproductibilité des measures de la tension arterielle et de la frequence cardiaque lors de l'épreuve d'effort. Arch Mal Coeur Vaiss (Suppl) 71:47–51

7. Dlin RA, Silverberg DS, Bar-Or O (1983) Follow-up of normotensive men with exaggerated pressure response to exercise. Am Heart J 106:316–320

8. Franz IW (1980) Differential antihypertensive effect of acebutolol and hy-drochlorothiazide/amiloride hydrochloride combination on elevated exer-cise blood pressure in hypertensive patients. Am J Cardiol 46:301–306

9. Franz I-W (1982) Assessment of blood pressure response during ergo-metric work in normotensive and hypertensive patients. Acta Med Scand Suppl 670:35–42

10. Franz I-W (1985) Ergometry in hypertensive patients. Implications for diagnosis and treatment. Springer, Berlin Heidelberg New York

11. Franz I-W (1993) Hypertonie und Herz. Springer, Berlin Heidelberg New York

12. Franz I-W, Lohmann FW (1978) Ergometry in the assessment of antihy-pertensive treatment. Dtsch Med Wochenschr 38:1487–1491

13. Franz I-W, Lohmann, FW (1982) Reproducibility of blood pressure mea-surements in hypertensives during and after ergometry. Dtsch Med Wo-chenschr 107:1379–1384

14. Franz I-W, Bartels F, Müller R (1982) Blood pressure response to ergo-metric work in normotensive subjects, aged 20–50 years. Z Kardiol 71:458–462

15. Franz I-W, Tönnesmann U, Erb D, Ketelhut R (1991) Impaired left ventri-cular function during exercise in hypertensives with normal coronary ar-teriograms. J Cardiovase Pharmacol 17 (Suppl 12):133–137

16. Franz I-W, Agrawal B, Wievel D, Ketelhut R (1992) Comparison of the antihypertensive effects of Carvedilol and Metoprolol on resting and ex-ercise blood pressure. Clin Invest 70:S53–S57

17. Gleichmann U (1984) Diskussionsbeitrag. In: Anlauf M, Bock KD (eds) Blutdruck unter körperlicher Belastung. Steinkopff, Darmstadt, pp 62–63

18. Gosse P, Campobello G, Aonizerate E, Roudaut R, Broustet LP, Dallochio M (1986) Left ventricular hypertrophy in hypertension: correlation with rest, exercise and ambulatory systolic blood pressure. J Hypertens Suppl 5:297–299

19. Gosse P, Durandet P, Roudant R, Broustet J-P, Dallochio M (1989) Prog-nostic value of blood pressure response during exercise in hypertensive patients. Fourth European Meeting on Hypertension, Milan (Abstract 307)

20. Gottdiener JS, Brown J, Zoltick J, Fletcher RD (1990) Left ventricual hy-pertrophy in men with normal blood pressure: relation to exaggerated blood pressure response to exercise. Am Intern Med 3:161–166

21. Gupta A, Manolio TA, Garrison RJ, Levy D (1992) Systolic blood pressure response to exercise predicts incident hypertension. The Framingham offspring study. J Am Coll Cardiol 19:86A
22. Heck H, Rost R, Hollmann W (1984) Normwerte des arteriellen Blutdruckverhaltens während fahrradergometrischer Belastung. In: Anlauf M, Bock KD (eds) Blutdruck unter körperlicher Belastung. Steinkopff, Darmstadt, pp 49–53
23. Hertzman PA (1993) Methods of blood pressure evaluation during exercise stress testing. In: Franz I-W (ed) Belastungsblutdruck bei Hochdruckkranken. Springer Berlin Heidelberg New York, pp 63
24. Hertzman PA (1995) Blood pressure response to exercise: diagnostic tool. Resident Staff Physician 41:23–28
25. Ketelhut RG, Ketelhut K, Franz I-W (1993) Blutdruckverhalten während Ergometrie in Abhängigkeit vom Trainingszustand und der Körperposition. In: Franz I-W (ed) Belastungsblutdruck bei Hochdruckkranken. Springer, Berlin Heidelberg New York, pp 28–35
26. Kjeldsen SZ, Mundal R, Sandrik L, Erikssen G, Thanlow E, Erikssen J (1994) Exercise blood pressure and fatal myocardial infarction. J Hypertens 12 (Suppl 3):77–82
27. Lassvik C (1978) Reproducibility of work performance and serical exercise in patients with angina pectoris. Scand J Clin Lab Invest 38:747–751
28. Leibel B, Kobrin I, Ben-Ishay D (1982) Exercise testing in assessment of hypertension. Br Med J 285:1535–1539
29. Löllgen H, Ulmer HV, Crean P (1988) Recommendations and standard guidelines for exercise testing. Eur Heart J 8 (Suppl 4):3–21
30. Lund-Johansen P (1967) Hemodynamics in essential hypertension. Acta Med Scand Suppl 482:1–11
31. Matthes D, Schütz P, Hüllemann KD (1978) Unterschiede zwischen indirekt und direkt ermittelten Blutdruckwerten. Med Klin 73:371–376
32. Millar-Craig MW, Balasubramamian V, Mann S, Raftery EB (1980) Use of graded exercise testing assessing the hypertensive patient. Clin Cardiol 3:236–241
33. Molineux D, Steptoe A (1988) Exaggerated blood pressure responses to submaximal exercise in normotensive adolescents with a family history of hypertension. Hypertension 6:361–366
34. Nathwani D, Reeves RA, Marquez-Julio A, Leenen FHH (1985) Left ventricular hypertrophy in mild hypertension: correlation with exercise blood pressure. Am Heart J 109:386–387
35. Patyna WD (1993) Belastungsblutdruck und Prognose nach Myokardinfarkt. In: Franz I-W (ed) Belastungsblutdruck bei Hochdruckkranken. Springer, Berlin Heidelberg New York, pp 171–182
36. Polonia J, Martins L, Bravo-Faria D, Macedo F, Continho J, Simones L (1992) Higher left ventricular mass in normotensives with exaggerated blood pressure responses to exercise associated with higher ambulatory blood pressure load and sympathetic activity. Eur Heart J 13 (Suppl A):30–36

37. Ren JF, Hakki AH, Kotler MN, Iskandrian AS (1985) Exercise systolic blood pressure: a powerful determinant of increased left ventricular mass in patients with hypertension. J Am Coll Cardiol 5:1224–1231
38. Rost R (1979) Kreislaufreaktion und -adaptation unter körperlicher Belastung. Osang, Bonn
39. Samek I, Betz P, Schnellbacher K (1984) Exercise testing in elderly patients with coronary artery disease. Eur Heart J 5 (Suppl G)
40. Sannerstedt R (1969) Hemodynamic findings at rest and during exercise in patients with arterial hypertension. Am J Med Sci 258:70–77
41. Wilson MF, Sung BH, Pincomb GA, Lovello WR (1990) Exaggerated pressure response to exercise in men at risk for systemic hypertension. Am J Cardiol 66:731–736
42. Wilson NV, Meyer BM (1981) Early prediction of hypertension using exercise blood pressure. Prev Med 10:62–66

β-Adrenergic Antagonists in the Management of Acute Myocardial Infarction

P. Soman, N. Lahiri, and A. Lahiri

Introduction

Despite significant advances in therapy, coronary artery disease is still the leading cause of mortality in the western world. Since the Goteborg metoprolol trial [1], several others have confirmed the beneficial effects of β-blockers in acute myocardial infarction. These range from a 13% reduction in mortality in the first 24 h after early intravenous β-blockade [2] to substantial reductions in mortality and morbidity resulting from chronic, long-term therapy in post-myocardial infarction patients. Although most of these trials were conducted in the pre-thrombolytic era, there is evidence to suggest that β-blockers, administered early in the post-myocardial infarction period offer significant benefits even to thrombolysed patients. The introduction of β-blockers with multiple actions such as carvedilol is likely to significantly extend their role in acute myocardial infarction and coronary artery disease.

The Pathophysiology of Acute Myocardial Infarction and Its Relevance to β-blockade

The transition from a slowly evolving atherosclerotic plaque to the acute coronary syndromes including unstable angina, non-Q wave myocardial infarction and Q wave myocardial infarction is usually precipitated by plaque rupture and the exposure of atherogenic substances that promote platelet activation and thrombus generation. The resultant thrombus interrupts blood flow, which, if complete and persistent, results in acute myocardial infarction and transmural myocardial necrosis. Lesser degrees and more transient obstruction cause non-transmural myocardial infarction and unstable angina [3, 4]. The interruption of this thrombotic process early in its evolution can potentially prevent the occurrence of acute myocardial infarction, or at least limit its extent.

There is a high incidence of ventricular arrhythmias in the early hours after acute myocardial infarction and 31%–50% of patients die from ventricular fibrillation before they reach hospital [2]. The ischaemic myocardium is very sensitive to the arrhythmogenic effects of catecholamines and free-radical release from the injured myocardium. After acute myocardial infarction, there is an increased concentration of circulating catecholamines and enhanced release of catecholamines from the nerve endings within the myocardium. Apart from its arrhythmogenic potential, this neurohormonal activation also has prognostic importance particularly in patients with left ventricular dysfunction, but also in those with acute myocardial infarction and normal left ventricular systolic function [5].

The extent of jeopardised myocardium (which includes necrosed, stunned and ischaemic myocardium) that remains after acute myocardial infarction determines both immediate and long-term prognosis. Necrosis of large areas of left ventricular myocardium can cause cardiogenic shock acutely, and predisposes to left ventricular failure and sudden death in the long term. Over a period of time, deleterious changes occur in the size, shape and thickness of left ventricular walls, which is collectively called "left ventricular remodelling" [4]. These changes consist of infarct expansion, ventricular dilatation and hypertrophy of the functioning myocardium, and are associated with a higher mortality rate and arrhythmias. Thus, measures to limit infarction will inhibit these changes.

Rationale for β-adrenergic Blockade After Acute Myocardial Infarction

β-Blockers reduce heart rate and blood pressure and therefore decrease myocardial oxygen demand. These properties could, at least theoretically, be used to advantage in the treatment of acute myocardial infarction, both in the short and long term. Experimental studies have shown that treatment with beta-blockers redistribute blood from the epicardium to the more ischaemic endocardium [6], protect against the deleterious effects of catecholamine toxicity to the myocyte, and favourably shift myocardial metabolism from free fatty acids to glucose [2]. In most patients presenting to hospital within the early hours after the onset of chest pain, the process of acute myocardial infarction will still be in evolution and further increases in the extent of myocardial necrosis may be expected to occur [7]. Therefore, to obtain maximum benefit, *β*-blockers must be instituted early after hospital presentation. Since effective blood levels are achieved only several hours after oral administration, the intravenous route has been recommended [8]. Thus early treatment with intravenous *β*-blockers would reduce ischaemic chest pain and ventricular arrhythmias, halt the evolution of infarction, limit infarct size, prevent re-infarctions and ultimately reduce mortality. However, an argument against early treatment is the fear of precipitating heart failure and complete heart block with the conventional *β*-blocker [9]. This dichotomy of risk and benefit has been the greatest hindrance to the widespread use of *β*-blockers early after acute myocardial infarction.

In the long term *β*-blockers could reduce angina, re-infarctions, arrhythmias, ventricular remodelling and the development of progressive heart failure [2, 10]. Therefore, the rationale and therapeutic objectives of the early and delayed institution of *β*-blockade after acute myocardial infarction are different and clinical trials examining each strategy have been performed.

The Evidence of Benefit from *β*-Blockers: Early Intravenous *β*-Blockade

Although the therapeutic objectives of *β*-blockade after acute myocardial infarction are multiple, the most important aim is to reduce mortality, both acutely and in the long term. However, the mortality benefit of any therapeutic intervention is difficult to demonstrate in any but the largest clinical trials. Although several trials of varying sizes have demonstrated similar percentage reductions in mortality from *β*-blockade after acute myocardial infarction, only the largest have been powered to produce statistically significant differences. Hence much of the mortality data has accrued from meta-analyses. Proof of reduction of ischaemic pain and in the number of completed infarctions by early intravenous β-blockade has been easier to come by. There is now convincing evidence that early β-blockade limits infarct size [11–14] and reduces ischaemic cardiac pain [15, 16]. An excellent overview of the available results indicate that the number of patients developing a definite infarct is reduced by about 13% by early β-blockade [2].

Much of the mortality data has come from the three largest trials, the Goteborg [1], First International Study of Infarct Survival (ISIS-1) [17] and the Metoprolol in Acute Myocardial Infarction (MIAMI) [18] trials. Although the probability of a beneficial effect of β-blockade after acute myocardial infarction was proposed as early as 1965 [19] the first large trial of early β-blockade after acute myocardial infarction was the Goteborg trial in 1981, where 1395 patients with known or suspected myocardial infarction were randomised to metoprolol (15 mg intravenously followed by 100 mg bd orally) or placebo which was started as soon as possible after the patients had arrived in hospital and continued for 90 days. Mortality was reduced by 36% in the metoprolol group over the 3-month period for which treatment was continued. However, the mean time from the onset of pain to β-blockade was 11.3 h, the mean reduction in creatine kinase rise was insignificant and the mortality benefit was evident later (weeks 2–13) rather than earlier. Therefore it is difficult to decide from this trial whether early intravenous administration provided any additional benefit over long-term oral β-blockers

The ISIS-I [17] included 16 027 patients randomised to intravenous atenolol or placebo within 5 h of onset of infarction and demonstrated a 14% reduction in vascular mortality at 1 week. The MIAMI [18] study with 5778 patients using metoprolol showed a 13% reduction in mortality over a 2-week treatment period (although this was not significant due to small sample size). All these trials pre-dated the use of thrombolysis.

The Thrombolysis in Myocardial Infarction (TIMI)-IIB trial [20] included a subgroup of 1434 thrombolysed patients in whom immediate versus deferred β-blockade was compared. The primary end point was global ejection fraction at hospital discharge, which was virtually identical in the two groups, and there was no difference in mortality. However, the study may not have been large enough to detect differences in mortality [2]. The combined end point of death or re-infarction at 6 weeks was significantly lower in patients who received β-blockers within 2 h of symptoms onset. There was a significantly lower incidence of re-infarction and recurrent chest pain at 6 days in the group which received intravenous metoprolol.

To date, more than 29 000 patients have been randomised in trials examining the mortality benefits of early intravenous β-blockade in acute myocardial infarction. Pooled analysis of data from all these clinical trials suggest that there is approximately a 13% reduction in the 7-day mortality, albeit with a wide 95% confidence interval of 3%–23% [2].

Long-Term β-Blockade

The major role of β-blockade, however, appears to be in the long-term treatment of post-myocardial infarction patients. Although more than 18 trials involving more than 20 000 patients have been reported, only a few of them were large enough to detect treatment effects on mortality [2].

The Norwegian Timolol trial [21] was the first one to convincingly demonstrate the benefits of long-term β-blockade after acute myocardial infarction. It included 1884 patients randomised to either oral timolol or placebo 7–28 days after acute myocardial infarction. After an average follow-up of 33 months, there was a 39% reduction in all-cause mortality in the timolol group, mainly due to reduced reinfarction and sudden deaths, which was evident irrespective of age and degree of risk. A 6-year follow-up of these patients suggested that the mortality benefit persisted in the timolol group. Olsson et al. [22] reported that, after a 3-year follow-up of patients given metoprolol after acute myocardial infarction, the overall benefits appear to increase with time and in those at increased risk (older patients with larger infarcts benefited more). The β-blocker Heart Attack Trial (BHAT) [23] randomised 3837 patients to oral propanolol or placebo 5–21 days after acute myocardial infarction. There was a 26% reduction in total mortality after 27 months, again largely due to a reduction in sudden death. In both these trials, mortality benefits were similar in both high and low risk groups, but the absolute benefits were higher in the high risk group. An overview of all the long-term trials suggests a mortality reduction of approximately 23% [2].

Mechanism of Mortality Reduction

Retrospective analysis of the ISIS data [17] suggests that much of the reduction in mortality occurs as a result of reduction in myocardial rupture in the first 2 days. Although this might largely explain the mechanism of mortality reduction, meta-analysis of all the available data also suggests a 15% reduction in the incidence of ventricular fibrillation and 18% reduction in re-infarction. The anti-arrhythmogenic effect may also contribute significantly towards the 32% reduction in sudden death seen with long-term β-blockade. However, β-blockers only have modest antiarrhythmic activity, and therefore their anti-ischaemic effects and reduction of sympathetic tone probably play a significant role [2].

Ancillary Properties of β-Blockers

Most of the evidence suggests that the benefits of these drugs are largely due to their β-blocking property rather than ancillary properties such as cardio-selectivity or membrane-selective activity, although post-infarction hypokalaemia may occur less frequently with non-selective β-blockers [24].

β-Blockade in the Context of Current Therapy for Acute Myocardial Infarction

The therapy of acute myocardial infarction has made dramatic strides in the past decade. Thrombolytic therapy has now become standard practice. Angiotensin-converting enzyme inhibitors are also widely used.

The majority of trials of β-blockers in acute myocardial infarction were conducted in the pre-thrombolytic era. The TIMI-IIB trial [20] compared intravenous and oral metoprolol in thrombolysed patients and found no difference in mortality, but reinfarctions were lower in the intravenously treated group. In the large studies of thrombolysis, the percentage of patients receiving β-blockade was low [25] and ranged from 6.4% in ISIS-2 [26] to 54% in AIMS [27]. Therefore, meaningful subgroup analysis was not possible. The small amount of data available on combination of the two therapies seems to suggest an additive effect.

When combined with thrombolytic therapy, β-blockers may offer several additional advantages to patients with myocardial infarction. Large trials have demonstrated an increase in early myocardial rupture after thrombolytic therapy [25]. β-Blockers reduce wall stress and may protect against myocardial rupture. Indeed, in the ISIS-1 trial [17] the mortality benefit of early intravenous atenolol was largely through reduction in cardiac rupture. The antifibrillatory effects of β-blockers may protect against reperfusion arrhythmias, and by reducing shear forces, they may reduce the incidence of intra-cranial cerebral haemorrhage as suggested by the TIMI II B results [20]. There is no evidence to suggest that combination therapy leads to an increased incidence of adverse events. In several studies combining atenolol or metoprolol with thrombolytic therapy [28–30], hypotension and other potential adverse events were uncommon in the β-blocker subgroup. The combination of β-blockers and angiotensin-converting enzyme inhibitors also seems to offer additive benefits. In the Survival And Ventricular Enlargement (SAVE) study [31] 1-year cardiovascular mortality, total cardiovascular mortality, incidence of severe heart failure and occurrence of the combined end-point were significantly lower in 789 patients who received a β-blocker in addition to angiotensin-converting enzyme inhibitors. The use of β-blockers was an independent predictor of prognosis [5]. A recent report on the SAVE study suggests that after acute myocardial infarction, the addition of β-blockers improves survival in patients with left ventricular dysfunction whose prognosis is also improved by the use of anglotensin-converting enzyme inhibitors [32]. However, despite this data, a significant number of patients with acute myocardial infarction, especially those with compromised cardiac

function, do not receive β-blockers. It is clear that many physicians are loath to use β-blockers in patients who would benefit
most from the treatment. The negative inotropic effect of conventional β-blockers is recognised and this inhibits their use in patients with heart failure.

Carvedilol

Carvedilol is a unique multiple action drug with non-selective
β-blocker and α-1-blocker effects [10]. It is also a potent anti-oxidant and may reduce damage caused by free radical generation
[33], and it alters lipid profile favourably by reducing LDL oxida-
tion [34]. We have had 15 years experience with carvedilol and
have shown its beneficial effects in angina [35], hypertension [36]
and ischaemic congestive heart failure [37]. Others have confirmed our findings in larger studies of congestive heart failure
[38]. A recent study has shown a large mortality benefit when carvedilol was added to conventional triple therapy for heart failure
management [39].

Animal studies have suggested that carvedilol may significantly
limit infarct size [40]. The Carvedilol Heart Attack Pilot Study
(CHAPS) [41] was performed at our centre in 151 consecutive patients with acute myocardial infarction who were randomised to
receive acute (intravenous) and long-term (6 months) oral treatment with either carvedilol or placebo. The data showed that carvedilol significantly reduced adverse cardiac events by 42%. Since
it has previously been established that intravenous carvedilol is
well tolerated by patients with congestive heart failure [42], patients with Killip classes I to III heart failure were included in the
CHAPS trial, unlike previous studies with β-blockers. Carvedilol
was well tolerated in the acute phase [43], and no patient was
withdrawn acutely due to worsening heart failure (Fig. 1). Indeed,
it has been suggested that to utilise the powerful anti-oxidant
properties of carvedilol [33] and its metabolites, the drug may
best be given prior to thrombolysis. This may reduce reperfusion
injury further. In the past carvedilol therapy has been shown to
reduce ventricular arrhythmias in a group of patients with various
cardiovascular diseases [44]. Also, there was a measurable reduc-

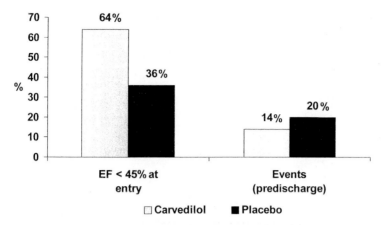

Fig. 1. The predischarge event rate in patients with ejection fraction (*EF*) <45% who were randomised to placebo or carvedilol in the CHAPS trial. Although 64% of patients with ejection fractions <45% received carvedilol, there was no increase in the incidence of adverse events in this group

tion in the incidence of sudden death in the US Carvedilol Heart Failure Study [39], and this may be of relevance to the management of myocardial infarction.

It is estimated that currently less than 50% of patients with acute myocardial infarction who are eligible for *β*-blockade actually receive these drugs whereas only 15% have contraindications for their use [25, 41]. This under-utilisation is largely due to fears of precipitating heart failure and conduction abnormalities. Although there was an increased incidence of heart failure, pacing and cardiogenic shock with intravenous compared to oral atenolol in GUST0 [9], this was not a randomised comparison. There were no significant differences in the incidence of atrioventricular blocks, congestive heart failure, or cardiogenic shock between the actively treated groups and control groups in the Goteborg [1] and MIAMI [18] trials, but the majority of these earlier studies excluded patients with heart failure. The *α*-blocking property of carvedilol produces rapid reduction in left ventricular filling pressure in heart failure patients (Fig. 2) [42]. Thus, patients with compromised left ventricular function can tolerate carvedilol better than conventional *β*-blocking drugs. It is likely that tolerance to *α*-blockade with carvedilol does not develop, since not only the

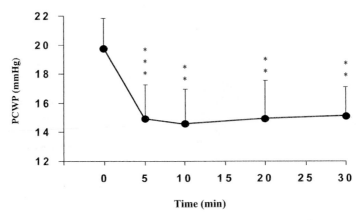

Fig. 2. The effect of intravenous carvedilol (2.5–7.5 mg) on pulmonary capillary wedge pressure (*PCWP*) in chronic heart failure: data from 17 patients with ischaemic cardiomyopathy with a mean ejection fraction (%) of 25±3. There was a significant reduction in PCWP with intravenous carvedilol which was maintained for 30 min. ** $p<0.005$; *** $p<0.0005$

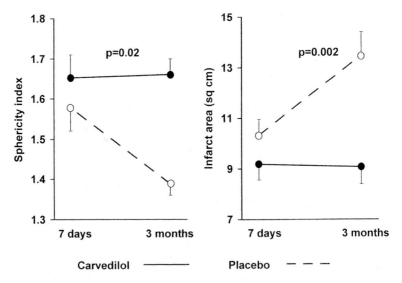

Fig. 3. The effect of carvedilol on the prevention of left ventricular remodelling after acute myocardial infarction: data from the CHAPS trial. The sphericity index was calculated as the ratio of the distances between the apical endocardium and the mitral annulus in the four-chamber view and between the septal and posterior wall endocardium in the short-axis view, and is a measure of left ventricular remodelling

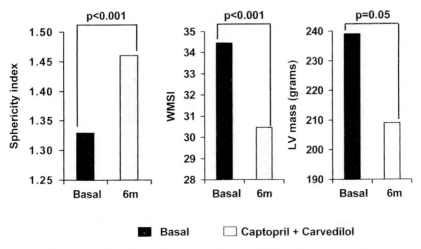

Fig. 4. The beneficial effect of combined carvedilol and captopril therapy on left ventricular (*LV*) remodelling in chronic congestive heart failure. The combined treatment produces significant reduction in left ventricular mass and improvement in sphericity index (indicating regression of remodelling). The reduction in the wall motion score index (*WMSI*) may represent an improvement in hibernating myocardium

drug is well tolerated during long-term treatment, but systemic vascular resistance remains low [37]. This may be reflected in some of the beneficial effects observed with carvedilol therapy [39, 46, 47].

Remodelling after acute myocardial infarction adversely affects prognosis. Data from the CHAPS trial suggests that carvedilol (in the absence of angiotensin converting enzyme inhibitors) may prevent or reverse ventricular remodelling after acute myocardial infarction [41]. New data from the CHAPS data base confirms that carvedilol prevents remodelling not only by reducing cardiac volume, but also by preventing infarct expansion and improving the sphericity index (calculated as the ratio of the distances between the apical endocardium and mitral annulus in the four chamber view, and the septal and posterior wall endocardium in the short-axis view) in patients with left ventricular dysfunction [48] (Fig. 3). Based upon the excellent pilot study CHAPS, larger clinical trials with carvedilol have now been set up, but they address the late phase of treatment following acute myocardial infarction. The question is: will carvedilol have additional benefit when added to angiotensin enzyme inhibitor treatment? Recent studies from our laboratory in congestive heart failure show a benefit of the combination of captopril and carvedilol, not only on remodelling but also on regional wall motion abnormality due to hibernating myocardium in patients with ischaemic cardiomyopathy [49] (Fig. 4).

Therefore carvedilol has an excellent safety profile in patients with acute myocardial infarction, even those with Killip I-III heart failure, and its beneficial properties may be of great relevance to the treatment of this common condition.

Summary

There is convincing evidence that β-blockers offer substantial benefits, both immediately and in the long term, after acute myocardial infarction. However, these drugs are currently under-utilised in this setting, primarily because of fears of precipitating heart failure or conduction abnormalities. The advent of newer agents with multiple actions, such as carvedilol, which appear to be safe even in patients with heart failure and have beneficial effects on heart failure, remodelling and free-radical suppression, should significantly promote the use of β-blockers in acute myocardial infarction.

References

1. Hialmarson A, Elmfeldt D, Herlitz J, et al. (1981) Effect on mortality of metoprolol in acute myocardial infarction. A double-blind randomised trial. Lancet ii:823–827.
2. Held PH, Yusuf S. (1993) Effects on β-blockers and calcium channel blockers in acute myocardial infarction. Eur Heart J 14(Suppl F):18–25
3. Fuster V, Badimon L, Badimon J, Cheserbo JH (1992) The pathogenesis of coronary artery disease and the acute coronary syndromes. N Engl J Med 326:310–316
4. Antman EM, Braunwald E (1997) Acute myocardial infarction. In: Braunwald E (ed) Heart disease. A textbook of cardiovascular medicine. Saunders, Philadelphia, pp 1184–1288

5. O'Rourke RA (1997) β-adrenergic blocking agents or angiotensin-converting enzyme inhibitors, or both, for post-infarction patients with left ventricular dysfunction. J Am Coil Cardiol 29:237–239

6. Buck JD, Hardman W, WarItier DC, et al. (1981) Changes in ischaemic blood flow distribution and dynamic severity of a coronary stenosis induced by β-blockade in the canine heart. Circulation 64:708–715

7. Yusuf S, Lopez P, Maddison A, Sleight P (1981) Variability of electrocardiographic and enzyme evolution of acute myocardial infarction in man. Br Heart J 43:271–280,

8. Rutherford JD, Singh BN, Ambler PK, Norris RM (1976) Plasma propanolol concentration in patients with angina and acute myocardial infarction. Clin Exp Pharmacol Physiol 3:297–304

9. Brener SJ, Cox JL, Pfisterer ME, Armstrong PW, Califf RM, Topol EJ, Gusto investigators (1995) The potential for unexpected hazard of intravenous β-blockade for acute myocardial infarction: results from the GUSTO trial. J Am Coll Cardiol 25 (Suppl):5A

10. Lahiri A (1996) Neurohormonal mechanisms in congestive heart failure and the role of drugs with multiple actions: a review of carvedilol. Am J Therapeutics 3:237–247

11. McIlmoyle L, Evans A, Mc Boyle CD, et al. (1982) Early intervention in mycoardical ischaemia. Br Heart J 47:189

12. Yusuf S, Ramsdale D, Peto R, Furse L, Bennett D, Bray C, Sleight P (1980) Early intravenous atenolol treatment in suspected acute myocardial infarction. Lancet ii:271–276

13. Peter T, Norris RM, Clarke ED (1978) Reduction of enzmye levels by propanolol after acute mayocardial infarction. Circulation 57:1091–1095

14. Norris RM, Sammel NL, Clarke ED, Brandt PWT (1980) Treatment of acute myocardial infarction with propanolol. Further studies on enzyme appearance and subsequent left ventricular function in treated and control patients with developing infarcts. Br Heart J 43:617–622

15. Herlitz J, Hjalmarson A, Holmberg S, et al. (1984) Effect of metoprolol on chest pain in acute myocardial infarction. Br Heart J 51:438–444

16. Ramsdale DR, Faragher EB, Bennett D, et al. (1982) Ischeamic pain relief in patients with acute myocardial infarction by intravenous atenolol. Am Heart 103:459–467

17. ISIS-I (First International Study of Infarct Survival) Collaborative Group (1986) Randomised trial of intravenous atenolol among 16 027 cases of suspected acute myocardial function. Lancet I:57–66

18. The MIAMI Trial Research Group (1985) Metoprolol in acute myocardial infarction (MIAMI). A randomised placebo-controlled international trail. Eur Heart J 6:199–226

19. Snow PJD (1965) Effect of propanolol in myocardial infarction. Lancet 2:551–553

20. Roberts R, Rogers WJ, Mueller HS, et al. (1991) Immediate versus deferred β-blockade following thrombolytic therapy in patients with acute

myocardial infarction. Results of the Thrombolysis In Myocardial Infarction (TIMI) II-B study. Circulation 83:422–437

21. Norwegian Multicentre Study Group (1981) Timolol-induced reduction in mortality and re-infarction in patients surviving acute myocardial infarction. N Engl J Med 304:801–807

22. Olsson G, Rehnqvist N, Sjorgren A, Erhardt L, Lundman T (1985) Long-term treatment with metoprolol after myocardial infarction: effect on 3-year mortality and morbidity. J Am Coll Cardiol 5:1428–1437

23. β-Blocker Heart Attack Trial Research Group (1982) A randomised trial of propanolol in patients with acute myocardial infarction. Mortality results. JAMA 247:1701–1714

24. Cleland JGF (1994) Overview of large clinical trials in patients with myocardial infarction. In: Cleland JGF, McMurray J Ray S (eds) Prevention strategies after myocardial infarction. Science Press Limited, London, pp 21–36

25. Olsson G, Held P (1993) Early intravenous β-blockade and thrombolytics in acute myocardial infarction. Am J Cardiol 71:156G–160G

26. ISIS-2 (Second International Study of Infarct Survical) Collaborative Group (1988) Randomised trail of intravenous streptokinase, oral aspirin, both or neither among 17 187 cases of suspected acute myocardial infarction: ISIS-2. Lancet ii:349–360

27. AIMS trial study group (1990) Long-term effects of intravenous anistreplase in acute myocardial infarction: final report of the AIMS study. Lancet 335:427–431

28. Risenfors M, Herlitz J, Berg CH, et al. (1991) Early treatment with thrombolysis and β-blockade in suspected myocardial infarction; results from the TEAHAT study. J Intern Med (Suppl 1):35–42

29. Vlay SC, Lawson WE (1988) The safety of combined thrombolysis and β-adrenergic blockade in patients with acute myocardial infarction: a randomised study. Chest 93:716–721

30. Green BKW, Gordon GD, Horak AR, Millar SRN, Crommerford PJ (1992) Safety of combined intravenous β-adrenergic blockade (atenolol or metoprolol) and thrombolytic therapy in acute myocardial infarction. Am J Coll Cardiol 69:1389–1392

31. Pfeffer MA, Braunwald E, Moye LA, et al. (1992) Effect of captopril on mortality and morbidity in patients with left ventricular dysfunction after myocardial infarction: results of the Survival and Ventricular Enlargement trial – the SAVE investigators. N Engl J Med 327:669–677

32. Vantripont P, Rouleau JL, Wun C-C, et al. (1997) Additive beneficial effects of β-blockers to angiotensin-converting enzyme inhibitors in the survival and ventricular enlargement (SAVE) study. J Am Coll Cardiol 29:229–236

33. Kramer JH, Weglicki WB (1996) A hydroxylated analogue of β-adrenoceptor antagonist, carvedilol, affords exceptional anti-oxidant protection to post-ischaemic rat hearts. Free Radic Biol Med 21:813–825

34. Hauf-Zachariou U, Widmann L, Zuelsdorf B, Hennig M, Lang PD (1993) A double-blind comparison of the effects of carvedilol and captopril on serum lipid concentrations in patients with mild to moderate essential hypertension and dyslipidaemia. Eur J Clin Pharmacol 45:95–100
35. Rodrigues EA, Lahiri A, Hughes LO, Kholi RS, Whittington JW, Raftery EB (1987) Anti-anginal efficacy of carvedilol: a new β-blocking drug with vasodilating activity. Am J Cardiol 58:916–921
36. Heber ME, Brigden GS, Caruana MP, Lahiri A, Raftery EB (1987) Carvedilol for systemic hypertension. Am J Cardiol 59:400–405
37. Dasgupta P, Broadhurst P, Raftery EB, Lahiri A (1990) Value of carvedilol in congestive heart failure secondary to coronoary artery disease. Am J Cardiol 66:1118–1123
38. Olsen SL, Gilbert EM, Renlund DG, Taylor DO, Yanowitz FD, Bristow MR (1995) Carvedilol improves left ventricular function and symptoms in chronic heart failure: a double-blind randomised study. A Am Coll Cardiol 25:1225–1231
39. Packer M, Bristwo MR, Cohn JR, et al. (1996) The effect of carvedilol morbidity and mortality in patients with chronic heart failure. N Engl J Med 334:1349–1355
40. Ruffolo RR Jr, Boyle DA, Brooks DP, Fuerstein GZ, Venuti RP, Lukas MA, Poste G (1992) Carvedilol: a novel cardiovascular drug with multiple actions. Cardiovasc Drugs Rev 10:127–157
41. Basu S, Raval U, Van der Does G, Bruckner T, Lahiri A (1997) Beneficial effects of intravenous and oral carvedilol treatment in acute myocardial infarction: a placebo controlled, randomised trial. Circulation 96:183–191
42. Dasgupta P, Broadhurst P, Lahiri A (1991) The effects of intravenous carvedilol, a new multiple action vasodilatory β-blocker in congestive heart failure. J Cardiovasc Pharmacol 18(Suppl 4):S 12–S 16
43. Basu S, Senior R, Kinsey C, Schaeffer S, Lahiri A (1997) Safety of early treatment with carvedilol in acute myocardial infarction with heart failure may be related to attenuation of left ventricular remodelling. Eur Heart J 18(Suppl):578
44. Senior R, Muller-Beckman B, Van der Does R, Dasgupta P, Lahiri A (1992) Effects of carvedilol on ventricular arrhythmia. J Cardiovasc Pharmacol 19(Suppl 1):S 117–S 121
45. Brand DA, Newcomer LN, Freiburger A, Tian H (1995) Cardiologists' practices compared with practice guidelines: uses of β-blockade after acute myocardial infarction. J Am Coll Cardiol 26:1432–1436
46. Olsen SL, Gilbert EM, Renlund DG, et al. (1991) Carvedilol improves left ventricular function in idiopathic dilated cardiomyopathy. Circulation 84(Suppl II):11–564
47. Bristow MR, Gilbert EM, Abraham WT, et al. for the MOCHA investigators (1996) Carvedilol produces dose-related improvements in left ventricular function and survival in subjects with chronic heart failure. Circulation 94:2807–2816

48. Senior R, Basu S, Lahiri A (1998) Carvedilol prevents remodelling in acute myocardial infarction with left ventricular dysfunction. J Am Coll Cardiol (in press)
49. Lahiri A, Senior R (1998) Imaging in ischaemic cardiomyopathy: therapeutic considerations. In: Zaret BL, Beller GA (eds) Nuclear cardiology. State of the art and future directions, 2nd edn. Mosby Yearbook, St. Louis (in press)

PART III

Angina Pectoris

β-Blocking Therapy in Patients with Unstable Angina

Andreas van de Loo

Introduction

Unstable angina is an acute coronary syndrome situated between chronic stable angina and acute myocardial infarction. The diagnosis depends on the presence of one or more characteristic facts from the patient's medical history: more intense or frequent anginal episodes with the background of pre-existing chronic stable angina; new onset of anginal symptoms within the last 4 weeks before presentation; or typical chest pain at rest or at minimal exer-

Table 1. Classification of unstable angina (from [2])

Class	Definition
I	New onset, severe or accelerated angina, less than 2 months' duration, severe or ocurring three or more times per day, or angina that is distinctly more frequent or precipitated by distinctly less exertion. No rest pain
II	Angina at rest, subacute. Patients with one or more episodes of angina at rest during the preceding month but not within the last 48 h
III	Angina at rest. Acute. Patients with one or more episodes at rest within the preceding 48 h
A	Secondary unstable angina Angina precipitated by a secondary cause: e.g., anemia, fever, infection, tachyarrhythmia, hypoxemia
B	Primary unstable angina
C	Postinfarction unstable angina
1	Absence of treatment or minimal treatment
2	Angina occurring in presence of standard conventional treatment
3	Angina occurring despite maximum antianginal treatment

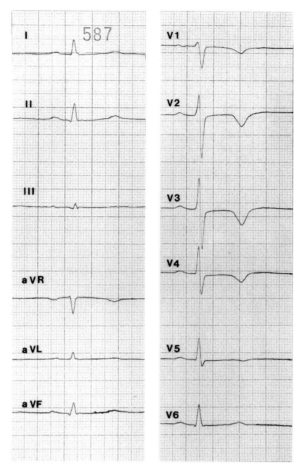

Fig. 1. Twelve-lead surface electrocardiogram of a female patient presenting with typical unstable angina

cise [1]. Braunwald [2] proposed a classification of angina in 1989 that reflects the most prominent characteristics of the patient's history (Table 1). Severity of anginal discomfort is described in classes I–III, and the clinical circumstances in which unstable angina occurs are classified A–C. The intensity of medical treatment at the time of onset of anginal pain is graded 1–3. It was the aim of this classification to define a common basis for both bedside and scientific evaluation of this heterogenous clinical entity.

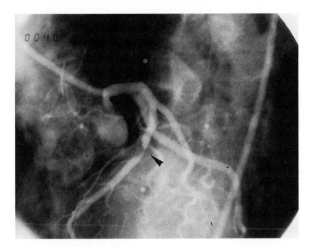

Fig. 2. Coronary angiogram of the same patient before acute percutaneous transluminal coronary angioplasty and stent implantation. Left anterior oblique view of the left coronary artery. *Arrow* pointing at severe proximal stenosis of the proximal left anterior descendent coronary artery

Patients with unstable angina present with a wide spectrum of clinical signs and symptoms. Typical anginal chest pain is frequently accompanied by tachycardia and hypertension as a consequence of the activation of the sympathetic autonomic system. Andrews et al. demonstrated the correlation between sympathetic activation as reflected by an increase in heart rate and the subsequent development of myocardial ischemia [3].

Characteristic changes in the 12-lead surface electrocardiogram are semimentation time (ST)-segment depression or transient ST-segment elevation (Fig. 1 and 2). Frequent ECG registrations are obligate during ischemic pain and after relief of the symptoms for risk stratification and optimal management. Recently published data from the electrocardiographic substudy of the Thrombolysis in Myocardial Ischemia (TIMI) III Registry define more precisely the significance of various alterations of repolarization in the surface ECG. The authors found during a 1-year follow-up period that initial ST-segment deviation (elevation or depression) of >0.5 mm and >1.0 mm and left bundle branch block were independent predictors of death and myocardial infarction. T-wave alteration does not seem to predict reliably an unfavorable outcome.

The authors conclude that clinicians should focus on subtle changes of the ST-segment when ruling out or confirming the diagnosis of unstable angina [4]. It is, however, very important to note that the clinical diagnosis of unstable angina is made by a precise characteristic patient history and examination. These electrocardiographic changes are not required for diagnosing unstable angina [2].

Pathophysiological Concept

The pathophysiological concept of unstable coronary syndromes is evolving continuously. The most frequent cause of unstable angina is the acute fissure of the fibrous cap of a chronic atherosclerotic lesion and consequent exposure of underlying thrombogenic tissue. Local intravascular thrombosis leads to intermittent severe reduction of coronary blood flow and consequent myocardial ischemia. However, angiographic studies after thrombolytic therapy for myocardial infarction revealed that many patients had intracoronary thrombosis without a significant stenotic lesion in the infarct-related artery [5, 6]. These observations led to scientific interest in the formation of atherosclerotic coronary plaques at the microscopic and molecular level. Today the differentiation between active or vulnerable and inactive or stable atherosclerotic plaque seems to be more appropriate [7]. A vulnerable plaque is not necessarily obstructing the coronary lumen and therefore not always detectable by conventional coronary angiography. In these lesions, microscopy detects a large eccentric lipid core and a very thin fibrous cap. The lipid core contains lipid-rich macrophages called foam cells [8]. The rupture of this fibrous cap exposes a highly procoagulant surface in contact with circulating blood [9]. Another relevant characteristic of the vulnerable plaque seems to be an infiltration of inflammatory cells, as demonstrated by Moreno et al. in a study comparing histological findings with coronary atherectomy specimens in patients with unstable angina and chronic stable angina [10]. In a postmortem study by van der Waal et al., an inflammatory infiltrate was a regular finding in coronary lesions that had acutely ruptured and caused fatal myocardial infarction [11]. The stable or inactive plaque is characterized by a small lipid core, a thick fibrous cap, and the lack of inflammatory cells [7]. Furthermore, the unstable coronary syndrome is characterized by increased platelet aggregability. Whether this is a primary cause of instability or a consequence of local coronary plaque rupture may be difficult to decide in individual patients. Platelet activation leads to release of thromboxane A and serotonine as very potent local vasoconstricting agents. Material from active atherosclerotic plaques expresses high amounts of endothelin-1, another potent vasoconstricting peptide [12]. Furthermore, endothelial dysfunction distal to coronary stenoses or occlusion contributes to the reduction of coronary blood flow and aggravation of anginal symptoms [13]. As a reflection of the local development of thrombosis in a coronary artery, it is possible to determine a systemic hypercoagulable state in patients suffering from acute onset of unstable angina. Markers of increased thrombin generation such as thrombin–antithrombin complex (TAT) and prothrombin fragment 1+2 (PF1+2) are elevated in these patients not only in the coronary veins but also in peripheral venous blood compared to patients with chronic stable angina [14, 15]. These data suggest that unstable angina should not be considered as a local coronary and myocardial problem but as a systemic condition that affects the entire organism.

Management of Unstable Angina

The optimal management of the unstable coronary syndrome requires precise and early diagnosis and prompt initiation of hemodynamic and arrhythmia monitoring. Immediate admission to a coronary care unit is generally recommended. The predominant goal of therapeutic interventions is the relief of anginal pain and prevention of evolving myocardial infarction [1]. The patient is positioned comfortably, oxygen is administered, and mild sedation is provided by diazepam or similar benzodiazepine derivatives. Intravenous morphine may be needed in some patients to effectively control anginal pain. Its analgetic and anxiolytic action is beneficial in this situation, and, furthermore, its peripherally vasodilating effect may reduce cardiac oxygen demand. The antithrombotic treatment is started as early as possible by intravenous (250–

500 mg) or oral (320–500 mg) aspirin. This drug has been investigated in numerous randomized prospective trials and has been proven to decrease the rate of developing myocardial infarction by up to 50% [16, 17, 18]. In 1988, Theroux et al. were able to show that early intravenous heparin could reduce the rate of developing myocardial infarctions in unstable angina compared to placebo. These results were confirmed by various other groups and today it is formally recommended to administer aspirin and heparin as early as possible in an unstable angina [19, 20, 21].

Nitrates are very effective in controlling anginal pain [1]. During the initial evaluation of the patient, sublingual nitrates are frequently used to differentiate unstable angina from myocardial infarction. Once the diagnosis has been established, 2–8 mg nitrate per minute are continuously infused for 24–48 h [22]. The dose should be continuously adjusted to the actual hemodynamic and anginal state of the patient.

As the acute and severe imbalance between cardiac oxygen supply and demand appears to be the most important factor in the progression of anginal pain and development of myocardial infarction, various therapeutic principles have been investigated to reduce cardiac oxygen demand. Sympathetic activity increases cardiac oxygen demand and impairs regional cardiac perfusion in ischemia. Therefore the use of β-blockers was an obvious therapeutic option. This group of drugs reduces myocardial oxygen demand by decreasing myocardial contractility, blood pressure, and heart rate. β-Blockers also decrease platelet aggregation [23] and they reduce shear stress, a significant contributor to increased thrombin generation in the unstable coronary syndrome [24]. Although the diagnosis of unstable coronary syndrome accounts for large numbers of hospital admissions in Western countries every year, β-receptor blocking therapy for unstable angina as a clinical entity has not been addressed in many prospectively designed, randomized studies as it has been in the case of patients with acute myocardial infarction. Our knowledge is therefore based on individual clinical experience and subgroup analyses of patients enrolled in the mega-trials directed to patients with suspected myocardial infarction. Various experimental studies demonstrated a reduction of infarct size even when a β-blocker was given hours after the onset of myocardial infarction [25, 26]. First clinical evidence for the beneficial effect of β-blocking agents was published as early as 1965 in the prethrombolytic period [27]. In this trial, patients with myocardial infarction or unstable angina were allocated to receive standard treatment or additional propranolol. Survival rate in the verum group was 84% as compared to the placebo-treated control group (64%). Norris et al. [28] conducted another early trial addressing β-blocking therapy in patients with unstable angina. These authors administered intravenous propanolol to 20 patients with unstable coronary syndrome defined as typical anginal chest pain without ECG changes suggesting myocardial infarction. Twenty-three patients fulfilling the same inclusion criteria served as the control group. Peak serum creatinine kinase was lower in the treatment group although the difference only reached borderline significance [28]. Yusuf et al. published a few years later a similarly designed study using atenolol as a β-blocker. In this study, 49% of those patients who received β-blocking therapy developed myocardial infarction during the follow-up phase compared to 66% of patients in the control group having received placebo [29]. The MIAMI (metoprolol in acute myocardial infarction) Trial [30] investigated early intravenous metoprolol as β-adrenoreceptor-blocking agent in patients with suspected acute myocardial infarction compared to placebo. Retrospective analysis of the subgroup of patients enrolled with unstable angina showed that 26% of those treated with metoprolol developed myocardial infarction compared to 31% in the placebo group. Subgroup analysis of these and various other larger intervention trials suggests that a reduction of the rate of developing myocardial infarction during follow-up is reduced by β-blocking therapy by up to 13% [31]. Today, early intravenous and oral β-blocker therapy has become a standard therapy for patients with unstable coronary syndromes and myocardial infarction [32, 33, 34]. Table 2 shows currently available studies on β-blockers in unstable angina. However, a surprising underuse of this therapeutic intervention which relieves anginal pain and reduces mortality has been reported from European and American authors for unstable angina and myocardial infarction [34, 35].

In two randomized prospective trials, the intravenous β-blocker esmolol was investigated in patients with unstable angina. Esmolol is characterized by a half-life of only a few minutes after intrave-

Table 2. β-Blockers in unstable angina: prospective clinical trials

Drug	Pa-tients	Dosage	Reference
Propranolol	20	0.1 mg/kg i.v.	[28]
Atenolol	NA	5–10 mg i.v. initial bolus, followed by 100 mg/day p.o.	Sleight, Am J Cardiol 1987
Metoprolol	79	2×100 mg/day p.o.	Lubsen, Circulation 1990
Metoprolol	NA	15 mg i.v. initial bolus, followed by 100–200 mg/day p.o.	Hjalmarsson, Lancet 1981
Esmolol	113	2–24 mg/min	[37]
Esmolol	23	10–20 mg i.v. initial bolus, followed by 2–24 mg/min	[36]
Carvedilol	116	50 mg/day p.o.	[42]

NA, no numbers available; data from subgroup analysis; i.v., intravenously; p.o., per os.

nous application. Wallis et al. [36] randomized patients to receive either an infusion of esmolol or oral propranolol as an adjunct to concomitant antianginal therapy. Both drugs reduced effectively heart rate, blood pressure, and ischemic episodes compared to a 24-h control period. In this small study (11 versus 12 patients), one adverse event occurred in each group. Discontinuation of the esmolol infusion was able to reverse hypotension. Severe drop in blood pressure in the propanolol group had to be treated by catecholamine infusion. In a large-scale prospectively randomized trial, Hohnloser et al. [37] compared esmolol to placebo in patients with unstable angina. The authors randomized 113 patients with an unstable coronary syndrome to receive either esmolol at a dose of 2–24 mg per minute or matching placebo. Esmolol induced a significant and persistent decline in heart rate and blood pressure. Predefined endpoints were myocardial infarction and the need for urgent revascularization. These endpoints occurred in nine patients of the control group and in three patients of the treatment group. Adverse effects occurred in both groups; esmolol induced significant bradycardia in 8% (0% in the placebo group) and severe hypotension in 12% (6%) of the patients. Pre-existing mild cardiac failure was documented in one patient of the esmolol group. All these adverse effects subsided after adjustment of the study dose [37].

These studies suggest that esmolol may be an interesting alternative drug to conventional *β*-blockers in unstable angina. However, experimental data show that esmolol has an additional cardio-depressant effect that is not explained by its *β*-receptor antagonism [38]. These data limit, in the authors' view, the clinical value of this cost-intensive drug in patients with unstable cardiac conditions.

The effect of a combined therapy with *β*-adrenoreceptor antagonists and calcium antagonists in unstable angina was addressed in the HINT (Holland Interuniversity Nifedipine/Metoprolol Trial) [39]. This multicenter randomized trial investigated oral nifedipine, metoprolol, and their combination in patients with unstable angina as admission diagnosis. The predefined clinical endpoint was recurrent ischemia. The authors found that in patients pretreated with oral *β*-blockers, the addition of oral nifedipine improves the clinical outcome. Orally applied metoprolol showed equally beneficial effects. Only in those patients on continuous *β*-blocker therapy the addition of nifedipine did improve outcome whereas the administration of nifedipine 6×10 mg daily alone showed a trend towards an unfavorable outcome – a finding that was confirmed by a controversially discussed recent meta-analysis on short-acting calcium antagonists in myocardial ischemia [40]. It has therefore been recommended to treat patients who are not free of anginal pain after effective *β*-blocker therapy with additional oral or intravenous nifedipine. In contrast to these early studies, the authors recommend the administration of slow-release formulations of this drug.

Carvedilol, a new *β*-receptor blocking agent, has additional peripheral vasodilating effects which result from a_1-adrenoreceptor blockade [41]. It is expected that besides the proven cardioprotective effect of this group of drugs, carvedilol might exert further beneficial effects by reducing cardiac afterload in patients with an unstable coronary syndrome. Experimental studies with this compound focused on myocardial salvage in the early treatment of myocardial infarction [41]. A similar positive effect might be expected in patients with unstable angina. Zehender et al. [42] conducted a double-blind, prospective placebo controlled study including 116 patients with unstable angina. The treatment group received carvedilol (50 mg per day orally) in addition to conventional therapy. The control group received matching placebo. The authors documented silent transitory ischemic episodes in the Holter ECG during a 48-h observation period. Carvedilol reduced frequency and duration of transitory ischemic episodes significantly compared to placebo. As in other studies [3], the onset of ischemia correlated with an increase in heart rate. The maximum protective effect was achieved 24 h after initiation of the carvedilol therapy. The investigators conclude that carvedilol as an adjunct to conventional therapy further reduces symptomatic and asymptomatic ischemic episodes as detected by ST-segment analysis compared to placebo [42]. However, as shown in the same study, potent β-blocking agents, particularly with additional vasodilating properties, require close hemodynamic and rhythm monitoring. Further investigations focusing on clinical endpoints like recurrent ischemia, myocardial infarction, or mortality are needed to finally evaluate this interesting pharmacological concept.

Conclusion

In conclusion, unstable angina is a severe clinical condition frequently equivalent to evolving myocardial infarction. The pathophysiological concept of this condition is progressing constantly and has lead to numerous studies investigating hemostatic markers as predictors for risk stratification and pharmacological interventions especially in the field of platelet aggregation. Acute management consists of various standardized anti-ischemic and antithrombotic agents. Early intravenous and oral β-adrenoreceptor blocking therapy in unstable angina has been demonstrated to be a potent medical strategy to relieve pain and to reduce the incidence of myocardial infarction. It is important to administer this drug as early as possible. Today, in the emergency setting 2–10 mg metoprolol intravenously or 0.5–1.0 mg i.v. of propranolol are recommended by an American expert panel, as published in 1994 [22]. This dose is adjusted to heart rate below 60 beats per minute and a systolic blood pressure below 110 mmHg. Absolute contraindications are heart block, chronic obstructive lung disease, and severe cardiac failure. Oral carvedilol seems to be a promising option in the therapy of patients with subacute unstable coronary syndrome as it adds the peripherally vasodilating effect to the proven *β*-blocking action. Its clinical relevance in the spectrum of pharmacological tools for the treatment of unstable angina needs to be evaluated by further prospective randomized trials.

Summary

Unstable angina is a frequent diagnosis at admission to hospital and a major cause of morbidity and mortality in Western countries. It is situated in the wide spectrum of coronary artery disease between chronic stable angina and acute myocardial infarction. The diagnosis is made predominantly on the basis of the patient's recent medical history. Intensity of anginal discomfort, clinical circumstances, and concomitant medical treatment are important aspects. Our understanding of the pathophysiology of unstable angina has changed considerably recently. It is seen as a syndrome with a local coronary thrombosis and complex alterations of the entire hemostatic system. In many patients it is not the chronic lumen-obstructing lesion that exacerbates to occlude the vessel but the acute rupture of a lipid-rich unstable coronary plaque. Therapeutic interventions aim to inhibit thrombus formation and to reduce cardiac oxygen demand. Essential immediate pharmacotherapy includes oral or intravenous aspirin and heparin.

Data from randomized prospective trials focusing on unstable angina are rare due to this heterogenous clinical entity. We therefore have to consider relatively small trials or subgroup analyses of the large studies on myocardial infarction. Intravenous application of *β*-receptor antagonists has been shown to reduce the rate of developing myocardial infarction significantly and to relieve anginal pain. Carvedilol, a *β*-receptor antagonist with additional vasodilating effect, was shown to reduce symptomatic and asymptomatic ischemic episodes in patients with unstable angina after oral application.

References

1. Baunwald E (ed) (1997) Heart disease, 5th edn, WB Saunders, Philadelphia
2. Braunwald E (1989) Unstable angina: a classification. Circulation 80:410–414
3. Andrews TC, Fenton T, Toyosaki N, Glasser SP, Young PM, Maccallum G, Gibson RS, Shook TL, Sone PH (1993) Subsets of ambulatory myocardial ischemia based on heart rate activity: circadian distribution and response to anti-ischemic medication. Circulation 88:92–100
4. Cannon CP, McCabe CH, Stone PH, et al. (1997) The electrocardiogram predicts one-year-outcome of patients with unstable angina and non-Q wave myocardial infarction: results of the TIMI III Registry ECG Ancillary Study. J Am Coll Cardiol 30:133–140
5. Hackett D, Davies G, Maseri A (1988) Pre-existing coronary stenoses in patients with first myocardial infarction are not necessarily severe. Eur Heart J 9:1317–1323
6. Ambrose JA, Tannenbaum MA, Alexopoulos D, Hjemdahl-Monsen CE, Leavy J, Weiss M, Borrico S, Gorlin R, Fuster V (1988) Angiographic progression of coronary artery disease and the development of myocardial infarction. J Am Coll Cardiol 12:56–62
7. Libby P (1995) Molecular bases of the acute coronary syndromes. Circulation 91:2844–2850
8. Libby P, Clinton SK (1993) The role of macrophages in atherogenesis. Curr Opin Lipidol 4:355–363
9. Wilcox JN, Smith KM, Schwartz SM, Gordon D (1989) Localization of tissue factor in the normal vessel wall and in the atherosclerotic plaque. Proc Natl Acad Sci USA 86:2839–2843
10. Moreno PR, Falk E, Placios IF, van der Loos CM, Newell JB, Fuster V, Fallon JT (1994) Macrophage infiltration in acute coronary syndromes: implication for plaque rupture. Circulation 90:775–778
11. Van der Waal AC, Becker AE, van der Loos CM, Das PK (1994) Site of intimal rupture or erosion of thrombosed coronary atherosclerotic plaques is characterized by an inflammatory process irrespective of the dominant plaque morphology. Circulation 89:36–44
12. Zeiher AM, Goebel H, Schächinger V, Ihling C (1995) Tissue endothelin-1 immunoreactivity in the active coronary atherosclerotic plaque. A clue to the mechanism of increased vasoreactivity of the culprit lesion in unstable angina. Circulation 91(4):941–947
13. Hirsh PD, Hillis LD, Campbell WB, Solymoss BC (1981) Release of prostaglandins and thromboxane into the coronary circulation in patients with ischemic heart disease. N Engl J Med 304:685–690
14. Merlini PA, Bauer KA, Oltrona L (1994) Persistent activation of coagulant mechanism in unstable angina and myocardial infarction. Circulation 90:61–66
15. Chesebro JH, Fuster V (1992) Thrombosis in unstable angina. N Engl J Med 327:192–196

16. The RISC Group (1990) Risk of myocardial infarction and death during treatment with low dose aspirin and intravenous heparin in men with unstable coronary artery disease. Lancet 336 f:827
17. Willard JE, Lange RA, Hillis LD (1992) The use of aspirin in ischemic heart disease. N Engl J Med 327:175
18. Antiplatelet Trialist's Collaboration (1994) Collaborative overview of randomized trials of antiplatelet therapy: I. Prevention of death, myocardial infarction and stroke by prolonged antiplatelet therapy in various categories of patients. Br Med J 308:81
19. Theroux P, Quimet H, McCans J, et al. (1988) Aspirin, heparin or both to treat unstable angina. N Engl J Med 319:1105
20. Theroux P, Waters D, Qiu S, et al. (1993) Aspirin versus heparin to prevent myocardial infarction during the acute phase of unstable angina. Circulation 88:2045–2048
21. Cohen M, Adams PC, Parry G, et al. (1994) Combination antithrombotic therapy in unstable rest angina and non-Q-wave infarction in nonprior aspirin users: primary end points analysis from the ATACS trial. Circulation 89:81
22. Braunwald E, Jones RH, Marks DB (1994) Diagnosing and managing unstable angina. Circulation 90:613–622
23. Winther K, Willich SN (1991) β_1-Blockade and acute coronary ischemia. Possible role of platelets. Circulation 84(Suppl VI):68–71
24. Hjemdahl P, Larsson PT, Wallen NH (1991) Effects of stress and *β*-blockade on platelet function. Circulation 84(Suppl VI)44–61
25. Miura M, Ganz W, Thomas R, Singh B, Sokol T, Shell WE (1966) Reduction of infarct size by propranolol in closed chest anaethetized dogs. Circulation II:159
26. Rasmussen MM, Reimer KA, Kloner RA, Jennings RB (1977) Infarct size reduction by propranolol before and after coronary ligation in dogs. Circulation 56:794–798
27. Snow PJD, Manc MD (1965) Effect of propranolol in myocardial infarction. Lancet 2:551–553
28. Norris RM, Clarke ED, Sammel NL, et al. (1978) Protective effect of propranolol in threatened myocardial infarction. Lancet 2:907–909
29. Yusuf S, Sleight P, Rossi P, et al. (1983) Reduction in infarct size, arrhythmias and chest pain by early intravenous beta blockade in suspected acute myocardial infarction. Circulation 67(6:Part 2):132–141
30. The MIAMI Trial Research Group (1985) Metoprolol in acute myocardial infarction (MIAMI). A randomized placebo controlled international trial. Eur Heart J 6:199–211
31. Yusuf S, Wittes J, Friedman L (1988) Overview of results of randomized clinical trials in heart disease: II. Unstable angina, heart failure, primary prevention with aspirin and risk factor reduction. JAMA 260:2259
32. Frishman WH (1983) Multifactorial actions of *β*-adrenergic blocking drugs in ischemic heart disease: current concepts. Circulation 67(6:Part 2):111–118

33. Frishman WH (1992) Beta-adrenergic blockers as cardioprotective agents. Am J Cardiol 70:2I–6I
34. Kennedy HL, Rosenson RS (1995) Physician use of beta-adrenergic blocking therapy: a changing perspective. J Am Coll Cardiol 26(2):547–552
35. Schuster S, Koch A, Burczyk U, et al. (1997) Frühbehandlung des akuten Myokardinfarkts: Umsetzung von Therapierichtlinien in den klinischen Alltag, MITRA-Pilotphase. Z Kardiol 86:273–283
36. Wallis DE, Pope C, Littman WJ, Scanlon PJ (1988) Safety and efficacy of esmolol for unstable angina pectoris. Am J Cardiol 62:1033–1037
37. Hohnloser SH, Meinertz T, Klingenheben T, Sydow B, Just H, for the European Esmolol Study Group (1991) Usefulness of esmolol in unstable angina pectoris. Am J Cardiol 67:1319–1323
38. Deegan R, Wood AJJ (1994) *β*-Receptor antagonism does not fully explain esmolol-induced hypotension. Clin Pharmacol Ther 56(2):223–228
39. Lubsen J, Tijssen JG (1987) Efficacy of nifedipine and metoprolol in the early treatment of unstable angina in the coronary care unit: findings from the Holland Interuniversity Nifedipine/Metoprolol Trial (HINT). Am J Cardiol 60:18A–25A
40. Furberg CD, Psaty BM, Meyer JV (1995) Nifedipine. Dose-related increase in mortality in patients with coronary heart disease. Circulation 92:1326–1331
41. Feuerstein GZ, Hamburger SA, Smith EF, Bril A, Ruffolo RR (1992) Myocardial protection with carvedilol. J Cardiovasc Pharmacol 19:138–141
42. Zehender M, Faber T, Schnabel P, Keck A, Jeron A, Greve B, Just H (1995) Benefits and hazards of carvedilol in unstable angina: a double blind placebo-controlled randomized study. Circulation 92(8):20

CHAPTER 6

Usefulness of β-Blockers in Sudden Cardiac Death

RALPH HABERL and GERHARD STEINBECK

Introduction

Sudden cardiac death continues to present an important ongoing problem, especially in association with severe underlying cardiac disease most commonly following myocardial infarction, and dilated cardiomyopathy. Less frequent causes include myocarditis, congenital long QT syndrome, mitral valve prolapse, sarcoidosis or hypertrophic obstructive cardiomyopathy. Sudden cardiac death can also be idiopathic, when a specific underlying disease cannot be found. The general aims of therapy depend on patient characteristics. In some cases, the aim is to prevent sudden cardiac death where it occurs without previously documented malignant ventricular arrhythmias; in other patients, the aim is to prevent recurrence in patients with previous episodes of such arrhythmias or resuscitated sudden cardiac death. Therapeutic strategies in the two types of patients will be different, although β-blockers have an important role to play in both cases. The aim of this chapter is to outline the usefulness of β-blockers in the prevention of sudden cardiac death in these two types of patient.

Classification of β-Blockers

In contrast to textbook classifications, electrophysiologists tend to characterise β-blockers according to their anti-arrhythmic properties (Table 1).

"Pure" β-blockers are those with no typical class I or class III actions; they do not prolong refractory time. Strictly speaking, they have no anti-arrhythmic effects; for example, they cannot

Table 1. The electrophysiologist's classification of β-blockers

I. Beta blockers without anti-arrhythmic action*
    1. "Pure" β-blockers
        With/without intrinsic sympathomimetic activity, β1 selective or not
    2. β- and α-receptor blockers
        Carvedilol
II. Anti-arrhythmics with β-blocking actions
    Including sotalol, propafenone, amiodarone

* Meaning no class I or III anti-arrhythmic action.

convert atrial fibrillation into sinus rhythm, or suppress accessory pathways. Pure β-blockers are also not pro-arrhythmic, apart from their ability to increase sinus bradycardia or promote the development of atrio-ventricular block. Carvedilol is an exception, as it has both beta- and alpha-blocking properties. Many still consider sotalol to be purely a β-blocker, but in its dl-form, it has strong class III effects with significant β-blocking (side) effects (d-sotalol is a pure class III anti-arrhythmic without β-blocker actions). Propafenone also has strong β-blocking activity and therefore has different anti-arrhythmic properties and pro-arrhythmic potential from other class IC anti-arrhythmics like flecainide. Amiodarone shows only small β-blocking effects together with strongly vasodilatatory action through α-blocking, and can therefore be used in patients with heart failure without much detrimental effect on cardiac function.

β-Blockers in the Primary Prevention of Sudden Cardiac Death

This section will discuss the use of β-blockers in patients who have never experienced sudden cardiac death nor had symptomatic sustained or non-sustained ventricular tachycardia documented, although ventricular extrasystoles or asymptomatic ventricular salvos might have been observed.

Arterial Hypertension

The Framingham study [33] indicated that arterial hypertension was an important factor in the development of coronary heart disease and sudden cardiac death. Treatment of hypertension with diuretics has been shown to reduce coronary events in elderly patients [10]; in contrast, angiotensin converting enzyme inhibitors, calcium antagonists and α-blockers have so far not been effective in reducing coronary events or sudden cardiac death. Several publications have reported that non-potassium sparing diuretics increase the risk of sudden cardiac death [26, 27, 50]; others do not agree [10]. β-blockers attenuate the increased risk of sudden cardiac death associated with non-potassium sparing diuretics (relative risk of 2.2 without versus 1.4 with β-blockers) [50]. It has been suggested that increased ventricular excitability can result from diuretic-induced potassium and magnesium loss [47]. The beneficial effects of β-blockers in this situation may be attributed to an anti-ischaemic component and a reduction in adrenaline-mediated intra-cellular potassium loss. In the MAPHY (Metoprolol Atherosclerosis Prevention in Hypertensives) study [39], five year mortality in patients treated with both metoprolol and thiazide diuretics was significantly lower than in those given only thiazide diuretics, an effect which could be primarily related to a 30% reduction in sudden cardiac death. Other studies have also demonstrated the benefit of β-blocker treatment in hypertensive patients [11, 17].

Acute Myocardial Infarction

Around 30–50% of patients die of ventricular fibrillation in the first hours after myocardial infarction, mostly before they have received medical help. More than 30 studies have shown that the early use of β-blockers (in the first 24 hours) reduces cardiac mortality and sudden cardiac death [65–67]. The ISIS (International Study of Infarct Survival)-1 study, which recruited more than 16 000 patients, showed that treatment with atenolol could reduce cardiovascular mortality in the first week by 14% [1]. At the time of this study, thrombolysis was not routinely given, and retrospective analysis of the data has shown that β-blocker treatment led to a reduction in myocardial rupture [6]; whereas sudden cardiac death was not separately evaluated. It has been calculated from pooled data that early β-blocker therapy in the acute phase after myocardial infarction could reduce mortality by about 15% in the first week [22]. The TIMI (Thrombolysis In Myocardial Infarction)-IIb trial demonstrated that early administration of β-blockers in combination with thrombolysis did not reduce the incidence of serious ventricular arrhythmias more than thrombolysis alone [46]. Hence, in the context of early reperfusion, there appears to be no advantage in administering β-blockers earlier rather than later (after more than one day). Early combination therapy using the negative chronotropes atenolol or alinidine together with alteplase thrombolysis in acute myocardial infarction reported similar short term results [21]. It has been suggested that the mechanisms of the beneficial effect of β-blockers in acute myocardial infarction include a redistribution of blood from the epicardium to the ischaemic endocardium, reduction in catecholamine-induced myocardial necrosis and beneficial effects on the metabolism of free fatty acids. The lowering of heart rate and blood pressure also decreases O_2 consumption and reduces myocardial wall tension, therefore minimizing infarct area. In many hospitals, these potentially beneficial effects of β-blockers are not fully utilized, especially in acute myocardial infarction patients on the brink of cardiogenic shock, as the worry is that their side effects of bradycardia and hypotension might be life-threatening in this situation [56].

Secondary Prevention after Myocardial Infarction

Beta blockers undoubtedly reduce the incidence of sudden cardiac death in the long term after myocardial infarction. Lipid lowering agents, acetyl salicylates and angiotensin converting agent inhibitors reduce the overall mortality after myocardial infarction, but could not reduce sudden cardiac death. Pooled data from about 20,000 patients on long term therapy with β-blockers after myocardial infarction has suggested a reduction in overall mortality of around 10%, with a reduction in that related to sudden cardiac death of between 32 and 50% [23, 25, 40, 44, 66]. The Norwegian

Timolol Trial and the β-Blocker Heart Attack Trial (BHAT) [42] investigated timolol or propranolol respectively and unanimously found a significant reduction in mortality of 3–6%. Although not explicitly investigated, a reduction in sudden cardiac death could be expected to have played an important role. Analysis of pooled data from five different studies where metoprolol was given in the long term after myocardial infarction showed that the reduction in overall mortality could mostly be attributed to a 40% reduction in sudden cardiac death [40]. Substances with intrinsic sympatho-mimetic activity (ISA) appear to act less through this mechanism [66].

The beneficial effect of β-blockers is particularly achieved by treating high risk patients with large infarcts, whereas patients with smaller infarcted areas and well-maintained left ventricular function benefit less or not at all. Hence, in clinical practice, the ongoing problem is that the patients with poor left ventricular function, where β-blockers might be thought to be relatively con-tra-indicated, stand to gain the most from treatment, which must be given at a sufficient therapeutic dose. A high number of side effects (particularly bradycardia, hypotension, orthostatic dysregu-lation, nightmares, impotence and bronchospasm) contributes to the fact that only about half the patients leave hospital with β-blocker treatment after myocardial infarction in Germany.

Risk stratification of post-infarct patients using analysis of late potentials is not adversely affected by β-blocker treatment, although this can alter measurements of heart rate variability.

Heart Failure

Severe underlying cardiac disease with heart failure is a strong risk factor for sudden cardiac death, irrespective of the heart dis-ease pathology itself. The ejection fraction is therefore one of the most useful predictors of sudden cardiac death. Cardiac failure in NYHA (New York Heart Association) class III or IV is associated with an overall mortality of approximately 50% over two years; in half of these through sudden cardiac death [49]. In these patient groups, anti-arrhythmic therapy with amiodarone does not reduce either the overall mortality, or sudden cardiac death. Studies investigating angiotensin converting enzyme inhibitors indicate a beneficial effect on overall mortality, but no improvement in rates of sudden cardiac death. Relatively recently, β-blockers have been used to good effect in patients with severe heart failure. Metoprolol (at gradually increasing doses of up to 100 to 150 mg daily) has been compared with placebo in 383 patients with heart failure secondary to dilated cardiomyopathy in NYHA class II or III who had ejection fractions of less than 40% [57, 58]. Although haemodynamic parameters and patient symptoms improved, and the time to needing heart transplant could be prolonged, the rate of sudden cardiac death was not altered (12/189 in the placebo group; 18/194 in the metoprolol group). In the Cardiac Insufficiency Bisoprolol Study (CIBIS), 641 patients were given bisoprolol (1.25 to 5 mg daily) or placebo in a randomised double-blind fashion [29]. Patients had NYHA class III or IV chronic heart failure with various underlying causes, and ejection fractions of less than 40%. At follow-up averaging 1.9 years, treatment with this β-blocker did not positively affect haemodynamics or sudden cardiac death (17 deaths in the placebo group; 15 deaths in the bisoprolol group), although there was a non-significant trend towards a reduced overall mortality in the active treatment arm. Retrospective analysis indicated that the mortality in patients with non-ischaemic dilated cardiomyopathy was significantly reduced by bisoprolol (42/187 deaths in patients in the placebo group; 18/151 deaths in patients treated with bisoprolol; no data on those with sudden cardiac death).

Carvedilol is in a special category of its own, as it is a non-selective beta-receptor antagonist, as well being able to block alpha-1 receptors. In contrast to other β-blockers, it also has anti-oxidant effects. Improvements in cardiac function and symptoms have been documented in patients with NYHA class II to IV heart failure and very low ejection fractions ($\leq$35%) with carvedilol treatment [36, 37]. In an Australian study of patients with NYHA class II or III, cardiac function was improved after six months, although patient symptoms appeared to be worsened [37]. Sudden cardiac deaths were not specifically investigated in this study. The United States study recruited 1,094 patients with chronic heart failure and ejection fractions of less than 35% who, according to current thinking, were already being optimally treated with diuretics and angiotensin converting enzyme inhibitors, some also with digoxin, hydralazine or nitrates [41]. Patients were randomised into a double blind trial of carvedilol (12.5 to 50 mg) versus placebo. Over six months follow-up, there were 31 deaths in the control group (7.8%; including 15 sudden cardiac deaths) and 22 in the carvedilol treated group (3.2%, of which 12 were sudden cardiac deaths). This was the first study to show that β-blocker therapy could reduce the mortality in severe heart failure. As a result of the positive result in favour of carvedilol, the study was discontinued early. It appears, however, to be too soon to suggest carvedilol as a routine treatment for severe heart failure. In particular, such therapy should only be undertaken in high risk patients with intensive monitoring, probably as an inpatient. Deaths have already been reported through aggravation of heart failure during the initiation of carvedilol treatment.

It is therefore clear that the only medical treatment that has shown any benefit in preventing sudden cardiac death in asymptomatic patients is β-blocker therapy. This is true whether the therapy is used for arterial hypertension, acute or chronic myocardial infarction or rarer diseases such as hypertrophic obstructive cardiomyopathy [15] or congenital long QT syndrome [13, 48]. A beneficial effect might be expected in patients with severe heart failure, especially those with non-ischaemic dilated cardiomyopathy. In contrast, anti-arrhythmics are not useful for reducing overall mortality [8, 30, 49]; some studies have been halted because of increased deaths in the treatment group [14, 59].

β-Blockers in the Secondary Prevention of Sudden Cardiac Death

In this section, the value of β-blocker therapy as secondary prevention against sudden cardiac death in patients who have had a symptomatic arrhythmic event or who have been resuscitated from sudden cardiac death will be discussed. β-blockers can have intrinsic anti-arrhythmic effects whether given alone or in combination with other anti-arrhythmics [3, 4, 24, 28, 35, 53, 55, 63] (Table 2).

Table 2. Use of β-block-
ers for primary preven-
tion of sudden cardiac
death in patients with-
out previous arrhythmic
events

- Arterial hypertension
- Myocardial infarction – acute phase
- Myocardial infarction – chronic phase
- Heart failure – varying pathogenesis
- Congenital long QT syndrome
- Hypertrophic (obstructive) cardiomyopathy

β-Blockers Given Alone as Anti-Arrhythmic Agent

β-blockers are the agent of choice for managing ventricular extrasystoles after myocardial infarction [18], in mitral valve prolapse
[34, 60, 68] or dilated cardiomyopathy. The advantage in these
cases is that pure β-blocker treatment is not associated with any
pro-arrhythmic effect, whereas more effective therapy of extrasystoles with class I or class III anti-arrhythmic drugs might worsen
prognosis, although the electrocardiogram will be improved. Class
I and III anti-arrhythmic drugs are therefore only indicated if
symptomatic therapy is specifically requested by patients or when
complications of tachycardic induced heart failure outweigh the
long term risks.

β-blockers have also been extensively tested in patients with
sustained symptomatic tachycardias without underlying cardiac
disease, where tachycardias were triggered by physical or psycho-
logical stress [5, 12, 16, 38]. This type of tachycardia often pre-
sents with left bundle branch block; suggesting right ventricular
origin. Inducibility through programmed ventricular stimulation
is often difficult or not possible; sometimes it is only achieved
after increasing heart rate with isoproterenol infusion (2–5 µg/
min raises the rate to about 120 beats/min). Metoprolol at a dose
of 200 mg daily can suppress clinical ventricular tachycardia in
about 50% of cases in the long term [5]. Other authors have also
reported good response to β-blockers in stress-induced ventricular
tachycardia [43, 53, 62]. Other therapeutic strategies include the
use of calcium antagonists, especially verapamil [2, 7, 19, 61, 64],
or combination therapy with β-blockers and anti-arrhythmics
[24].

The use of β-blockers alone for sustained ventricular arrhythmias in patients with proven underlying cardiac disease (particu-

larly after myocardial infarction or cardiomyopathy) is more controversial. A retrospective study has shown that patients resuscitated after sudden cardiac death have a better prognosis with β-blocker therapy [20]. The gold standard for deciding on the best therapy for symptomatic sustained ventricular tachycardia is invasive electrophysiological testing. However, it has not yet been proven that this costly procedure where anti-arrhythmics are serially tested really reduces the incidence of recurrent tachycardias or sudden cardiac death. Our group has therefore undertaken a prospective trial in 170 patients with varying underlying cardiac diseases who have had suppressible sustained ventricular tachycardia, ventricular fibrillation or syncope, and underwent electrophysiological testing [51]. If the arrhythmias were inducible, patients were randomised either to serial anti-arrhythmic testing (class I anti-arrhythmic drugs with metoprolol, sotalol and amiodarone) or to metoprolol alone (100–200 mg/day), patients in whom the tachycardias were not inducible received empirical treatment with metoprolol at this dose. After an average follow-up of 23 months, 44 patients had recurrent symptomatic ventricular tachycardia, and 27 had died of sudden cardiac death. There was no difference in these complications between groups with serial testing or empirical metoprolol. However, effective anti-arrhythmic treatment could only be found in 21% of patients who were serially tested (6 of the 29 patients in this group died during follow-up), and those who continued to be inducible had a poor prognosis (21 of 32 patients died). At the time of the study, they could not yet be treated with an implantable defibrillator. Despite this, in half these high risk patients treated with β-blockers alone for two years there was no recurrence of arrhythmia or sudden cardiac death. This raises the question of whether anti-arrhythmic agents can improve overall prognosis at all. It could be argued that a positive response to serial anti-arrhythmic testing could be a result of selecting those patients who would have had a good response anyway, irrespective of administration of any anti-arrhythmic agent. If this is true, then a patient who appears to have a suppressible arrhythmia with a particular anti-arrhythmic should have a good prognosis even when the agent is later stopped. A study to address this point is currently underway within our group (the Anti-arrhythmic Drugs Improve Outcome Study

(ADIOS) [52]). Patients with spontaneous sustained and inducible ventricular tachycardia suppressible with anti-arrhythmic drugs are eligible for the study. They all receive an implantable defibrillator, and are randomised to be further treated with the "effective" anti-arrhythmic agent or not. Initial results suggest that rates of complications are comparable in both groups (Hoffmann et al., American Heart Association meeting 1997). The conclusions from the ESVEM (Electrophysiology Study Versus Electrocardiographic Monitoring) study, where sub-group analysis found sotalol therapy to be superior to class I anti-arrhythmics in patients with symptomatic ventricular tachycardia and syncope (although the primary endpoint was investigation of Holter testing versus ventricular stimulation), [31, 45] must now be interpreted in the light of these results. As there was no control group in the ESVEM study, it is difficult to make any real conclusions about the true efficiency of anti-arrhythmic therapy.

β-Blockers in Combination with Anti-Arrhythmic Therapy

Combining anti-arrhythmic and β-blocker treatments can be considered when, as in the case of sotalol, the anti-arrhythmic to be used does not already possess a significant degree of β-blocking action per se. Cobb et al. found that in survivors of sudden cardiac death, there was no significant difference between patients treated with and without concomitant propranolol therapy [9]. Concomitant β-blocker therapy has been shown to be particularly useful in problematic patients with markedly reduced left ventricular function and sustained arrhythmias. This is remarkable, as this combines anti-arrhythmic agents which are mostly negatively inotropic (apart from amiodarone), with drugs which further worsen heart function. However, patients with poor left ventricular function and arrhythmias often have high catecholamine levels which could benefit from β-blocker treatment. In a retrospective study of 32 patients with ventricular fibrillation or sustained ventricular tachycardias, and very poor left ventricular function (ejection fraction of below 40%), Brodski showed that additional β-blocker therapy improved exercise tolerance and that the therapy could be continued in the long-term without significant side effects [4]. In a similar patient group with severely reduced left ventricular function (ejection fraction <45%) and symptomatic sustained ventricular arrhythmias, Szabo found that administration of β-blockers was associated with lower cardiac mortality and a reduced risk of sudden cardiac death [54]. In multi-variate analysis, very low ejection fraction (≤27%), lack of β-blocker therapy and severe heart failure were the strongest predictors of sudden cardiac death. Hence, concomitant β-blocker therapy often appears to be useful and well tolerated by patients with severe left ventricular dysfunction. In clinical practice, medical therapy is limited to patients in whom a procedure (for example, ablation or surgery) directed against the underlying cause is not possible, or where a spontaneous arrhythmic event would not be so life-threatening that a primary implantable cardiac defibrillator should be sited. In addition, certain patients who have had a defibrillator implanted will need anti-arrhythmics as well, to reduce the frequency of discharging events. In complicated cases with recurrent arrhythmias, we combine amiodarone with a β-blocker and a class I anti-arrhythmic (for example mexitil). Clearly the medical management of such a patient will be initiated only in a specialist centre for the treatment of arrhythmias.

β-blockers also have their place as additional therapy in patients with implantable defibrillators. Firstly, they are indicated when an inappropriate sinus or atrial tachycardia leads to ventricular rates approaching the trigger rate of the defibrillator: β-blockers help to reduce the number of inappropriate shocks. Secondly, patients with implantable defibrillators treated with β-blockers receive significantly fewer "appropriate" shocks as a result of recurrent arrhythmias [32], although this has only been shown in a small number of patients and deserves further investigation.

Hence β-blockers have an important role to play in the primary prevention of sudden cardiac death in patients who are up until now asymptomatic, as well as in the management of patients with previous arrhythmic events. To date, despite competition from other classes of agent, they are the only medical treatment whose use in preventing sudden cardiac death is of value. This can be related to their anti-ischaemic, anti-arrhythmic and anti-fibrillatory actions.

References

1. Anderson S, Blanski L, Byrd RC, Das G, Engler R, Laddu A, Lee R, Rajfer S, Schroeder J, Steck JD, et al. (1986) Randomised trial of intravenous atenolol among 16027 cases of suspected acute myocardial infarction: ISIS-1. First International Study of Infarct Survival Collaborative Group. Lancet 2:57-66

2. Belhassen B, Shapira I, Pelleg A, Copperman I, Kauli N, Laniado S (1984) Idiopathic recurrent sustained ventricular tachycardia responsive to vera-pamil: an ECG-electrophysiologic entity. Am Heart J 108:1034-1037

3. Brodsky MA, Allen BJ, Baron D, Chesnie BM, Abate D, Thomas R, Henry WL (1986) Enhanced survival in patients with heart failure and life-threatening ventricular tachyarrhythmias. Am Heart J 112:1166-1172

4. Brodsky MA, Allen BJ, Bessen M, Luckett CR, Siddiqi R, Henry WL (1988) Beta-blocker therapy in patients with ventricular tachyarrhyth-mias in the setting of left ventricular dysfunction. Am Heart J 115:799-808

5. Brodsky MA, Orlov MV, Allen BJ, Orlov YS, Wolff L, Winters R (1996) Clinical assessment of adrenergic tone and responsiveness to beta-block-er therapy in patients with symptomatic ventricular tachycardia and no apparent structural heart disease. Am Heart J 131:51-58

6. Buck JD, Hardman HF, Warltier DC, Gross GJ (1988) Mechanisms for the early mortality reduction produced by beta-blockade started early in acute myocardial infarction: ISIS-1. ISIS-1 (First International Study of Infarct Survival) Collaborative Group. Lancet 1:921-923

7. Buxton AE, Waxman HL, Marchlinski FE, Simson MB, Cassidy D, Joseph-son ME (1983) Right ventricular tachycardia: clinical and electrophysio-logic characteristics. Circulation 68:917-927

8. Cairns JA, Connolly SJ, Roberts R, Gent M (1997) Randomised trial of outcome after myocardial infarction in patients with frequent or repeti-tive ventricular premature depolarisations: CAMIAT. Canadian Amiodar-one Myocardial Infarction Arrhythmia Trial Investigators. Lancet 349:675-682

9. Cobb LA, Weaver WD, Fahrenbruch CE, Hallstrom AP, Copass MK (1992) Community-based interventions for sudden cardiac death. Impact, limitations, and changes. Circulation 85:I98-102

10. Cohn JN, Johnson G, Ziesche S, Cobb F, Francis G, Tristani F, Smith R, Dunkman WB, Loeb H, Wong M, et al. (1991) Prevention of stroke by antihypertensive drug treatment in older persons with isolated systolic hypertension. Final results of the Systolic Hypertension in the Elderly Program (SHEP). SHEP Cooperative Research Group. JAMA 265:3255-3264

11. Dahlof B, Lindholm LH, Hansson L, Schersten B, Ekbom T, Wester PO (1991) Morbidity and mortality in the Swedish Trial in Old Patients with Hypertension (STOP-Hypertension). Lancet 338:1281-1285

12. DiCarlo LA, Susser F, Winston SA (1990) The role of beta-blockade therapy for ventricular tachycardia induced with isoproterenol: a prospective analysis. Am Heart J 120:1347–1355
13. Eldar M, Griffin JC, Van Hare GF, Witherell C, Bhandari A, Benditt D, Scheinman MM (1992) Combined use of beta-adrenergic blocking agents and long-term cardiac pacing for patients with the long QT syndrome. J Am Coll Cardiol 20:830–837
14. Epstein AE, Bigger JT, Wyse DG, Romhilt DW, Reynolds Haertle RA, Hallstrom AP (1991) Events in the Cardiac Arrhythmia Suppression Trial (CAST): mortality in the entire population enrolled. J Am Coll Cardiol 18:14–19
15. Fananapazir L, McAreavey D. Hypertrophic cardiomyopathy: evaluation and treatment of patients at high risk for sudden death. Pacing Clin Electrophysiol 20:478–501
16. Fei L, Statters DJ, Hnatkova K, Poloniecki J, Malik M, Camm AJ (1994) Change of autonomic influence on the heart immediately before the onset of spontaneous idiopathic ventricular tachycardia. J Am Coll Cardiol 24:1515–1522
17. Fletcher A, Beevers DG, Bulpitt C, Butler A, Coles EC, Hunt D, Munro F, Newson RB, O'Riordan PW, Petrie JC, et al. (1988) Beta adrenoceptor blockade is associated with increased survival in male but not female hypertensive patients: a report from the DHSS Hypertension Care Computing Project (DHCCP). J Hum Hypertens 2:219–227
18. Frishman WH, Furberg CD, Friedewald WT (1984) Beta-adrenergic blockade for survivors of acute myocardial infarction. N Engl J Med 310:830–837
19. Gill JS, Blaszyk K, Ward DE, Camm AJ (1993) Verapamil for the suppression of idiopathic ventricular tachycardia of left bundle branch block-like morphology. Am Heart J 126:1126–1133
20. Hallstrom AP, Cobb LA, Yu BH, Weaver WD, Fahrenbruch CE (1991) An antiarrhythmic drug experience in 941 patients resuscitated from an initial cardiac arrest between 1970 and 1985. Am J Cardiol 68:1025–1031
21. Heidbüchel H, Tack J, Vanneste L, Ballet A, Ector H, Van DE (1994) Significance of arrhythmias during the first 24 hours of acute myocardial infarction treated with alteplase and effect of early administration of a beta-blocker or a bradycardiac agent on their incidence. Circulation 89:1051–1059
22. Held P, Yusuf S (1989) Early intravenous beta-blockade in acute myocardial infarction. Cardiology 76:132–143
23. Hinkle LE, Thaler HT (1982) A randomized trial of propranolol in patients with acute myocardial infarction. I. Mortality results. JAMA 247:1707–1714
24. Hirsowitz G, Podrid PJ, Lampert S, Stein J, Lown B (1986) The role of β-blocking agents as adjunct therapy to membrane stabilizing drugs in malignant ventricular arrhythmia. Am Heart J 111:852–860

25. Hjalmarson A, Elmfeldt D, Herlitz J, Holmberg S, Malek I, Nyberg G, Ry-
    den L, Swedberg K, Vedin A, Waagstein F, Waldenstrom A, Waldenstrom
    J, Wedel H, Wilhelmsen L, Wilhelmsson C (1981) Effect on mortality of
    metoprolol in acute myocardial infarction. A double-blind randomised
    trial. Lancet 2:823–827
26. Hoes AW, Grobbee DE, Peet TM, Lubsen J (1994) Do non-potassium-
    sparing diuretics increase the risk of sudden cardiac death in hyperten-
    sive patients? Recent evidence. Drugs 47:711–733
27. Jazayeri MR, Van Wyhe G, Avitall B, McKinnie J, Tchou P, Akhtar M
    (1982) Multiple risk factor intervention trial. Risk factor changes and
    mortality results. Multiple Risk Factor Intervention Trial Research Group.
    JAMA 248:1465–1477
28. Jazayeri MR, van Wyhe G, Avitall B, McKinnie J, Tchou P, Akhtar M
    (1989) Isoproterenol reversal of antiarrhythmic effects in patients with
    inducible sustained ventricular tachyarrhythmias. J Am Coll Cardiol
    14:705–711
29. Jazayeri MR, van Wyhe G, Avitall B, McKinnie J, Tchou P, and Akhtar M
    (1994) A randomized trial of beta-blockade in heart failure. The Cardiac
    Insufficiency Bisoprolol Study (CIBIS). CIBIS Investigators and Commit-
    tees. Circulation 90:1765–1773
30. Julian DG, Camm AJ, Frangin G, Janse MJ, Munoz A, Schwartz PJ, Simon
    P (1997) Randomised trial of effect of amiodarone on mortality in pa-
    tients with left-ventricular dysfunction after recent myocardial infarction:
    EMIAT. European Myocardial Infarct Amiodarone Trial Investigators.
    Lancet 349:667–674
31. Klein RC (1993) Comparative efficacy of sotalol and class I antiarrhyth-
    mic agents in patients with ventricular tachycardia or fibrillation: results
    of the Electrophysiology Study Versus Electrocardiographic Monitoring
    (ESVEM) Trial. Eur Heart J 14(Suppl H):78–84
32. Leclercq JF, Leenhardt A, Coumel P, Slama R (1992) Efficacy of beta-
    blocking agents in reducing the number of shocks in patients implanted
    with first-generation automatic defibrillators. Eur Heart J 13:1180–1184
33. Levy D, Wilson PW, Anderson KM, Castelli WP (1990) Stratifying the pa-
    tient at risk from coronary disease: new insights from the Framingham
    Heart Study. Am Heart J 119:712–717
34. Martini B, Basso C, Thiene G (1995) Sudden death in mitral valve pro-
    lapse with Holter monitoring-documented ventricular fibrillation: evi-
    dence of coexisting arrhythmogenic right ventricular cardiomyopathy. Int
    J Cardiol 49:274–278
35. Meredith IT, Broughton A, Jennings GL, Esler MD (1991) Evidence of a
    selective increase in cardiac sympathetic activity in patients with sus-
    tained ventricular arrhythmias. N Engl J Med 325:618–624
36. Olsen SL, Gilbert EM, Renlund DG, Taylor DO, Yanowitz FD, Bristow MR
    (1995) Carvedilol improves left ventricular function and symptoms in
    chronic heart failure: a double-blind randomized study. J Am Coll Cardi-
    ol 25:1225–1231

37. Olsen SL, Gilbert EM, Renlund DG, Taylor DO, Yanowitz FD, Bristow MR (1995) Effects of carvedilol, a vasodilator-beta-blocker, in patients with congestive heart failure due to ischemic heart disease. Australia-New Zealand Heart Failure Research Collaborative Group. Circulation 92:212–218

38. Olshansky B, Martins JB (1987) Usefulness of isoproterenol facilitation of ventricular tachycardia induction during extrastimulus testing in predicting effective chronic therapy with beta-adrenergic blockade. Am J Cardiol 59:573–577

39. Olsson G, Tuomilehto J, Berglund G, Elmfeldt D, Warnold I, Barber H, Eliasson, K, Jastrup B, Karatzas N, Leer J, et al. (1991) Primary prevention of sudden cardiovascular death in hypertensive patients. Mortality results from the MAPHY Study. Am J Hypertens 4:151–158

40. Olsson G, Wikstrand J, Warnold I, Manger Cats V, McBoyle D, Herlitz J, Hjalmarson A, Sonneblick EH (1992) Metoprolol-induced reduction in postinfarction mortality: pooled results from five double-blind randomized trials. Eur Heart J 13:28–32

41. Packer M, Bristow MR, Cohn JN, Colucci WS, Fowler MB, Gilbert EM, Shusterman NH (1996) The effect of carvedilol on morbidity and mortality in patients with chronic heart failure. U.S. Carvedilol Heart Failure Study Group. N Engl J Med 334:1349–1355

42. Peters RW, Muller JE, Goldstein S, Byington R, Friedman LM (1989) Propranolol and the morning increase in the frequency of sudden cardiac death (BHAT Study). Am J Cardiol 63:1518–1520

43. Podrid PJ, Lown B (1982) Pindolol for ventricular arrhythmia. Am Heart J 104:491–496

44. Pratt CM, Francis MJ, Luck JC, Wyndham CR, Miller RR, Quinones MA (1981) Timolol-induced reduction in mortality and reinfarction in patients surviving acute myocardial infarction. N Engl J Med 304:801–807

45. Reiffel JA (1996) Implications of the Electrophysiologic Study versus Electrocardiographic Monitoring trial for controlling ventricular tachycardia and fibrillation. Am J Cardiol 78:34–40

46. Roberts R, Rogers WJ, Mueller HS, Lambrew CT, Diver DJ, Smith HC, Willerson JT, Knatterud GL, Forman S, Passamani E, et al. (1991) Immediate versus deferred beta-blockade following thrombolytic therapy in patients with acute myocardial infarction. Results of the Thrombolysis in Myocardial Infarction (TIMI) II-B Study. Circulation 83:422–437

47. Siegel D, Hulley SB, Black DM, Cheitlin MD, Sebastian A, Seeley DG, Hearst N, Fine R (1992) Diuretics, serum and intracellular electrolyte levels, and ventricular arrhythmias in hypertensive men. JAMA 267:1083–1089

48. Singh B, Al Shahwan SA, Habbab MA, Al Deeb SM, Biary N (1993) Idiopathic long QT syndrome: asking the right question. Lancet 341:741–742

49. Singh SN, Fletcher RD, Fisher SG, Singh BN, Lewis HD, Deedwania PC, Massie BM, Colling C, Lazzeri D (1995). Amiodarone in patients with congestive heart failure and asymptomatic ventricular arrhythmia. Sur-

vival Trial of Antiarrhythmic Therapy in Congestive Heart Failure. N Engl J Med 333:77–82

50. Siscovick DS, Raghunathan TE, Psaty BM, Koepsell TD, Wicklund KG, Lin X, Cobb L, Rautaharju PM, Copass MK, Wagner EH (1994) Diuretic therapy for hypertension and the risk of primary cardiac arrest. N Engl J Med 330:1852–1857

51. Steinbeck G, Andresen D, Bach P, Haberl R, Oeff M, Hoffmann E, von Leitner ER (1992) A comparison of electrophysiologically guided antiarrhythmic drug therapy with beta-blocker therapy in patients with symptomatic, sustained ventricular tachyarrhythmias. N Engl J Med 327:987–992

52. Steinbeck G, Haberl R, Hoffmann E (1996) Electropharmacological drug testing. In: Saksena S, Lüderitz B (eds): Interventional electrophysiology. A Textbook. Futura Publishing Company, Armonk, NY pp 203

53. Sung RJ, Shen EN, Morady F, Scheinman MM, Hess D, Botvinick EH (1983) Electrophysiologic mechanism of exercise-induced sustained ventricular tachycardia. Am J Cardiol 51:525–530

54. Szabo BM, Crijns HJ, Wiesfeld AC, van Veldhuisen DJ, Hillege HL, Lie KI (1995) Predictors of mortality in patients with sustained ventricular tachycardias or ventricular fibrillaion and depressed left ventricular function: importance of beta-blockade. Am Heart J 130:281–286

55. Taylor RR, Halliday EJ (1965) Beta-adrenergic blockade in the treatment of exercise-induced paroxysmal ventricular tachycardia. Circulation 32:778–781

56. van de Werf F, Janssen L, Brzostek T, Mortelmans L, Wackers FJ, Willems GM, Heidbuchel H, Lesaffre E, Scheys I, Collen D, et al. (1993) Short-term effects of early intravenous treatment with a beta-adrenergic blocking agent or a specific bradycardiac agent in patients with acute myocardial infarction receiving thrombolytic therapy. J Am Coll Cardiol 22:407–416

57. Waagstein F, Bristow MR, Swedberg K, Camerini F, Fowler MB, Silver MA, Gilbert EM, Johnson MR, Goss FG, Hjalmarson A (1993) Beneficial effects of metoprolol in idiopathic dilated cardiomyopathy. Metoprolol in Dilated Cardiomyopathy (MDC) Trial Study Group. Lancet 342:1441–1446

58. Waagstein F, Caidahl K, Wallentin I, Bergh CH, Hjalmarson A (1989) Long-term beta-blockade in dilated cardiomyopathy. Effects of short- and long-term metoprolol treatment followed by withdrawal and readministration of metoprolol. Circulation 80:551–563

59. Waldo AL, Camm AJ, de Ruyter H, Friedman PL, MacNeil DJ, Pauls JF, Pitt B, Pratt CM, Schwartz PJ, Veltri EP. Effect of d-sotalol on mortality in patients with left ventricular dysfunction after recent and remote myocardial infarction. The SWORD Investigators. Survival With Oral d-Sotalol. Lancet 348:7–12

60. Werdan K, Muller U (1989) Mitral valve prolapse and mitral valve prolapse syndrome. Internist 30:475–482

61. Woelfel A, Foster JR, McAllister RG, Simpson RJ, Gettes LS (1985) Efficacy of verapamil in exercise-induced ventricular tachycardia. Am J Cardiol 56:292–297
62. Woelfel A, Foster JR, Simpson RJ, Gettes LS (1984) Reproducibility and treatment of exercise-induced ventricular tachycardia. Am J Cardiol 53:751–756
63. Woosley RL, Kornhauser D, Smith R, Reele S, Higgins SB, Nies AS, Shand DG, Oates JA (1979) Suppression of chronic ventricular arrhythmias with propranolol. Circulation 60:819–827
64. Wu D, Kou HC, Hung JS (1981) Exercise-triggered paroxysmal ventricular tachycardia. A repetitive rhythmic activity possibly related to afterdepolarization. Ann Intern Med 95:410–414
65. Yusuf S (1987) Interventions that potentially limit myocardial infarct size: overview of clinical trials. Am J Cardiol 60:11A–17A
66. Yusuf S, Peto R, Lewis J, Collins R, Sleight P (1985) Beta blockade during and after myocardial infarction: an overview of the randomized trials. Prog Cardiovasc Dis 27:335–371
67. Yusuf S, Wittes J, Friedman L (1988) Overview of results of randomized clinical trials in heart disease. I. Treatments following myocardial infarction. JAMA 260:2088–2093
68. Zuppiroli A, Mori F, Favilli S, Barchielli A, Corti G, Montereggi A, Dolara A (1994) Arrhythmias in mitral valve prolapse: relation to anterior mitral leaflet thickening, clinical variables, and color Doppler echocardiographic parameters. Am Heart J 128:919–927

β-Blocking Agents in Patients with Coronary Artery Disease and Myocardial Infarction

Michael Christ and Martin Wehling

Introduction

Myocardial infarction (MI) and ischemic stroke are regarded as the most frequent causes of death in Germany (Statistisches Bundesamt 1997), the United States (Kannel and Thom 1994) and other western industrialized countries. Costs of primary and secondary health care due to morbidity of cardiovascular diseases, not to mention mortality have led to the search for potent and effective treatment strategies to diminish coronary and cerebrovascular handicaps, and to prevent new ones.

In the 1980s, β-adrenergic receptor blockers ("β-blockers") became the most popular form of antihypertensive therapy after diuretics. Their popularity reflects their effectiveness in the prevention of ischemic stroke in hypertensives and virtual absence of serious side effects (Joint National Committee 1993). In addition, β-blockers have been investigated in the prevention of myocardial infarction: first clinical studies for secondary prevention of myocardial infarction were carried out in the mid 1960s with propranolol (Propranolol Study Group 1966), for which a beneficial prognostic action was postulated (Snow 1966). Only small numbers of patients were included in these trials in the 1960s and 1970s; thus, results have been heterogeneous, though promising (for a review see Yusuf et al. 1985, Hjalmarson and Olsson 1991; Hampton 1994). In the early 1980s, large, prospective, and randomized clinical trials were designed to prove the beneficial effects of β-blockers in the secondary prevention of myocardial infarction, as postulated some 20 years earlier (Multicenter International Group 1977; Hjalmarson et al. 1981; Norwegian Multicentre Study Group 1981; BHAT 1982; Salathia et al. 1985; Boissel et al.

Table 1. Trials with early and late study entry are separated. ISA, intrinsic sympathomimetic activity; MSA, membrane-stabilizing activity; p-value, computed for chi-square test comparing the proportion of deaths in each

Trial	β-Blocker	Dose	Duration of treatment	Selectivity	ISA	MSA
• Early entry (<24 h)						
Barber et al. 1976	Practolol	300 mg bd	2 y	β_1	+	–
Salathia et al. 1985	Metoprolol	15 mg iv+ 200 mg po/day	1 y	β_1	–	(+)
Hjalmarson et al. 1981	Metoprolol	15 mg iv+ 100 mg bid po	3 mo	β_1	–	(+)
Wilcox et al. 1980a	Propranolol or atenolol	40 mg tid 50 mg bd	1 y	β_1, β_2 β_1	– –	+ –
Anderson et al. 1979	Alprenolol	5–10 mg iv+ 200 mg bid po	1 y	β_1, β_2	+	+
Wilcox et al. 1980b	Oxprenolol	40 mg tid	6 wk	β_1, β_2	+	(+)
Basu et al. 1997	Carvedilol	2.5 mg iv+ 12.5–25 mg bid	6 mo	β_1, β_2	–	(+)
• Late entry (>24 h)						
Boissel et al. 1990	Acebutolol	200 mg bid	∼10.5 mo	β_1	+	(+)
Multicenter International Group 1977	Practolol	200 mg bid	1–3 y	β_1	+	–
Olsson et al. 1985	Metoprolol	100 mg bid	3 y	β_1	–	(+)
Lopressor Study Group 1987	Metoprolol	100 mg bid	1 y	β_1	–	(+)
Australian and Swedish Pindolol Study Group 1983	Pindolol	15 mg/d	2 y	β_1, β_2	++	(+)
Wilhemlsson et al. 1974	Alprenolol	400 mg/d	2 y	β_1, β_2	+	+
CPRG 1981	Oxprenolol	40 mg bd	∼2 mo	β_1, β_2	+	(+)
Taylor et al. 1982	Oxprenolol	40 mg bid	mean 4 y	β_1, β_2	+	(+)
E.I.S. 1984	Oxprenolol	160 mg bid	1 y	β_1, β_2	+	(+)
Baber et al. 1980	Propranolol	40 mg tid	3–9 mo	β_1, β_2	–	+
Hansteen et al. 1982	Propranolol	40 mg qid	1 y	β_1, β_2	–	+
BHAT 1982	Propranolol	60–80 mg tds	∼2 y	β_1, β_2	–	+
Norwegian Multicentre Study Group 1981	Timolol	10 mg bid	∼17 mo	β_1, β_2	–	(+)
Julian et al. 1982	Sotalol	320 mg/d	1 y	β_1, β_2	–	–
Total (pooling of data)						

group. E.I.S, European Infarction Study; BHAT, Beta-Blocker Heart Attack Trial; CPRG, Coronary Prevention Research Group

Basic data from trials (deaths/total patients) (%)		Statistics		
Allocated control	Allocated β-blocker	Relative risk	95% CI	p-value
47/147 (31.3)	41/151 (27.2)	0.85	0.60–1.21	0.36
43/364 (11.8)	**27/391 (6.9)**	**0.58**	**0.37–0.92**	**0.02**
62/697 (8.9)	**40/698 (5.7)**	**0.64**	**0.44–0.94**	**0.02**
12/122 (9.8)	28/251 (11.2)	1.13	0.84–1.52	0.70
64/242 (26.2)	60/238 (25.2)	0.95	0.70–1.29	0.76
6/154 (3.9)	8/151 (5.3)	1.36	0.80–2.30	0.56
3/71 (4.2)	2/75 (2.7)	0.63	0.11–3.61	0.60
34/309 (11.0)	**17/298 (5.7)**	**0.52**	**0.30–0.90**	**0.02**
78/1533 (5.1)	**48/1520 (3.2)**	**0.62**	**0.44–0.88**	**0.007**
31/147 (21.1)	25/154 (16.2)	0.77	0.48–1.24	0.28
62/1200 (5.2)	65/1195 (5.4)	1.05	0.90–1.25	0.77
47/266 (17.7)	45/263 (17.1)	0.97	0.67–1.40	0.87
14/116 (12.1)	7/114 (6.1)	0.55	0.24–1.30	0.17
3/134 (2.2)	6/174 (3.4)	1.54	0.40–5.98	0.53
48/471 (10.2)	60/632 (9.5)	0.93	0.65–1.34	0.70
45/880 (5.1%]	57/858 (6.6)	1.30	0.89–1.89	0.17
27/365 (7.4)	28/355 (7.9)	1.07	0.82–1.38	0.80
37/282 (13.1)	25/278 (9.0)	0.69	0.43–1.10	0.12
188/1921 (9.8)	**138/1916 (7.2)**	**0.74**	**0.60–0.91**	**0.004**
152/939 (16.2)	**98/945 (10.4)**	**0.64**	**0.51–0.81**	**0.0002**
52/583 (8.9)	64/873 (7.3)	0.82	0.58–1.17	0.27
1055/10 943 (9.6)	**889/11 540 (7.7)**	**0.80**	**0.73–0.87**	**<0.0001**

1990; see Table 1). Critical reviews and meta-analyses discussing more than 30 randomized studies with β-blockers (small and large ones) were in favor of these drugs for treatment of coronary artery disease after myocardial infarction (Yusuf et al. 1985; Hampton 1994): studies in more than 20000 patients have shown a rate of reinfarction reduced by $\sim 27\%$, total mortality reduced by $\sim 22\%$ and sudden death reduced by $\sim 32\%$ (Yusuf et al. 1988). In addition to late onset and chronic therapy with β-blockers, results of large, randomized studies (Hjalmarson et al. 1981; ISIS 1986) were in favor of their intravenous administration very early in myocardial infarction, which was reflected in the recommendations of the American College of Cardiology and the American Heart Association (ACC/AHA Task Force 1996).

This overview predominantly focusses on results of *long-term* trials in secondary prevention of myocardial infarction. In addition to a critical reevaluatation of these "ancient" trials, newer compounds of this group will be introduced and their effectiveness with regard to secondary prevention of coronary artery disease discussed.

For the choice of a particular β-blocker, the following questions should be answered:

- Which group of patients with coronary artery disease benefits most? Should every patient without contraindications be treated with β-blockers?
- Are there any results in prospective clinical trials which indicate the preference of particular compounds?
- What is the optimal dose of β-blockers?
- Which controlled clinical studies demonstrate beneficial effects of β-blockers in combination with additional modern drug therapies such as thrombolysis and angiotensin-converting-enzyme (ACE) inhibition?

Myocardial Infarction and Experimental Effects of β-Blockade

In addition to an increased risk for reinfarction (GISSI-1 1987), patients who survive myocardial infarction have a high risk of sudden and non-sudden death presumably due to life-threatening arrhythmias and chronic, progressive cardiac failure (Yusuf et al. 1988). During acute coronary syndromes, some 30%–50% of patients die early from ventricular fibrillation (Armstrong et al. 1972; Pedoe et al. 1975). Short- and long-term prognosis of survivors, who reach emergency care alive, depends on the amount of remaining viable myocardium (Sobel et al. 1972): patients with large areas of infarction tend to develop impaired left ventricular function and develop cardiogenic shock, late ventricular arrhythmias, or secondary ventricular fibrillation (Page et al. 1971; Thompson et al. 1979). Activation of the sympatho-adrenergic system secondary to myocardial infarction and heart failure has been demonstrated to be an indicator of emerging complications (Rouleau et al. 1993, 1994): in addition to increases in myocardial oxygen demand (Maroko et al. 1971) and increased susceptibility of the myocardium to ventricular arrhythmias (Dhurandhar et al. 1971; Campbell et al. 1981) by sympatho-adrenergic activation (Vantrimpont et al. 1997), decreases in oxygen supply, e.g., via hypoxemia (Radvany et al. 1975), anemia (Yoshikawa et al. 1973) or hypoglycemia (Libby et al. 1975), have been held responsible for fatal events during and after myocardial infarction.

By counteracting the direct adverse effects of catecholamines, *β*-blockers may reduce myocardial workload, and hence myocardial oxygen demand, by lowering heart rate and blood pressure (Kjekshus 1986). In addition, these agents may reduce arrhythmic death (Yusuf et al. 1985; Hampton 1994; Kennedy et al. 1994); they act indirectly by reducing free fatty acid levels and by shifts of the myocardial metabolism from fatty acids to glucose, thereby further decreasing oxygen demand (Mueller and Ayres 1977; Simonsen and Kjekshus 1978). Moreover, *β*-blockade can reduce catecholamine levels (Mueller and Ayres 1980) and produces a beneficial redistribution of blood flow in the myocardium (Pitt and Craven 1970). On that theoretical basis, drug therapy aimed at reducing sympatho-adrenergic effects should be beneficial with regard to cardiac fatalities as demonstrated in experimentally induced myocardial infarction (Opie and Thomas 1976; Reimer et al. 1976; Waldenstrom et al. 1979): indeed, *β*-blockers have been shown to reduce infarct size (measured by indirect indexes such as enzyme levels or electrocardiographic changes), decrease myocardial wall stress, and prevent cardiac rupture (Yusuf et al. 1983,

1985). In addition, a significant reduction of ventricular arrhythmias was found (Rossi et al. 1983; ISIS-1 1988). All these mechanisms are expected to reduce early and late mortality, reinfarction, ventricular fibrillation and chronic heart failure.

Pharmacological Properties of β-Adrenergic Receptor Antagonists

The β-adrenergic receptor antagonists are effective in reducing severity and frequency of angina pectoris due to fixed, morphological coronary stenosis (Dargie et al. 1996; Pepine et al. 1994; Portegies et al. 1994) by reducing myocardial oxygen demand. Although propranolol has been the agent evaluated most extensively, most β-blockers appear to be equally effective in the treat-ment of exertional angina. The effectiveness of β-blockers is mostly attributable to a net reduction of myocardial oxygen consumption at rest and during exercise (Hoffman and Lefkowitz 1995).

All β-adrenergic receptor antagonists are competitive, partial or complete antagonists which inhibit the interaction of epinephrine, norepinephrine and other sympathomimetics with β-adrenergic receptors. Since compounds have been developed with different affinities for the various subtypes of these receptors, selective interference with responses caused by stimulation of the sympathetic nervous system can be evoked. Propranolol, the prototype of β-blockers, was introduced during the early 1960s (Black and Stephenson 1962). Propranolol is devoid of agonist activity and demonstrates a nonselective inhibition of the β-adrenoceptor subtypes. Subsequent research generated additional antagonists that can be distinguished by following properties (see also Table 1): relative affinity for β_1- and β_2-receptors, intrinsic sympathomimetic activity, additional blockade of α_1-subtype receptors, differences in lipid solubility, capacity to induce vasodilation, and general pharmacokinetic properties. Some of these distinguishing characteristics are likely to have clinical significance (see below) and may be used to guide the appropriate choice of a β-receptor blocker in an individual patient. However, one has to keep in mind that "cardioselective" does not mean "cardiospecific": selectivity for any subtype of adrenoceptor depends on the dosage used and the route of administration. Thus, a β_1-selective antagonist such as metoprolol can still aggravate asthma, especially allergic asthma. When discussing possible beneficial effects of β_1-selective antagonists (e.g., metoprolol or atenolol), one has to remember that large doses have been given in controlled clinical trials, whereas much lower doses are often used in clinical practice (Viskin et al. 1995; Viskin and Barron 1996).

β-Blockers for the Primary Prevention of Myocardial Infarction

In contrast to studies with estrogens and aspirin (Physician's Health Study Group 1989; Bronner et al. 1995; Fuster and Chesebro 1995; Rich-Edwards et al. 1995; Maron 1996) aimed at the primary prevention of cardiovascular events (e.g., ischemic stroke, myocardial infarction), no trials with β-blockers have been carried out to answer this question. Thus, most knowledge is derived from large randomized blood pressure trials where the actions of β-blockers have been studied.

However, unlike trials on secondary prevention of myocardial infarct (MI), the primary goal of these trials was to demonstrate a beneficial effect of blood pressure control (Hampton 1994). Trials can be categorized into three types: (a) trials demonstrating favorable effects of any form of active treatment versus placebo, (b) trials comparing various treatment regimens, and (c) trials comparing two or more individual antihypertensive drugs. Except for type c, the benefit of β-blockers cannot be derived from studies aimed at blood pressure control as opposed to studies on the secondary prevention of myocardial infarction.

While in the Oslo (Helgeland 1980) and Australian studies (The Australian therapeutic trial in mild hypertension 1980) and in the MRFIT (Grimm et al. 1985) and SHEP (1991) β-blockers were added if diuretic treatment proved insufficient (propranolol, pindolol or atenolol), in the Study of Coope and Warrender (metoprolol; 1985) and in the Swedish STOP trial (atenolol or propranol; Dahlof et al. 1991) a β-blocker was used as first – line therapy. In one trial (IPPPSH 1985), the inclusion of oxprenolol, a compound without or with only detrimental effects on secondary prevention of myocardial infarction, has been compared with other antihypertensive drug regimens. In the MRC-1 trial (Medical Research Council 1985) propranolol was compared with a diuretic, as was atenolol in the MRC-2 trial (MRC Working Party 1992). In the HAPPHY trial (Wilhelmsen et al. 1987), two different β-blockers, atenolol and metoprolol, could be used to control high blood pressure. While the β-blocker group was compared with diuretics, atenolol was not compared with metoprolol (Wilhelmsen et al. 1987). Adding to the difficulty in generating general recommendations, in some trials only men were studied, while in others only elder patients (ranging from 60 to 70 years of age) were enrolled. It is very difficult to clearly establish the extent of benefit in relation to these different antihypertensive treatments at all. However, in the EWPHE (European Working Party 1985), SHEP (SHEP 1991), STOP (Dahlof et al. 1991) and MRC-2 (MRC Working Party 1992) studies, in which only elderly hypertensives were included, a reduction of the incidence of myocardial infarction has been demonstrated for β-blockers (range of risk reduction: 13%–27%). However, these studies do not support specific recommendations as to the use of particular β-blockers. Since in one study diuretics have shown even more favorable effects in the reduction of the cardiac fatality rate (Wilhelmsen et al. 1987) – an advantage which has not been explained until today – the clinician's choice is triggered by additional specific group effects, e.g., side effects in relation to the patient's individual demands.

In summary, at present there are no large trials demonstrating a specific favorable effect of β-blockers on the primary prevention of myocardial infarction. Results from large hypertension trials give evidence that β-blockers reduce overall mortality in hypertensives (presumably via decreasing blood pressure), but specific beneficial effects of β-blockers on myocardial infarction have been shown in only a few trials. Some trials showed no effects on infarction rates (MRC-2), and others even suggest that diuretics should be preferred in hypertensives for the prevention of myocardial infarction (Wilhelmsen et al. 1987). In addition, there is currently no evidence from controlled trials that any β-blocker should be preferred over another.

β-Blockade for Secondary Prevention of Myocardial Infarction

The following section gives a comprehensive overview of large intervention trials on the chronic effects of β-blockade in the treatment of coronary artery disease.

Since the late 1960s randomized trials have been conducted to test the hypothesis that β-blockers may provide a beneficial effect in the secondary prevention of myocardial infarction (Balcon 1966). From the mid 1960s to 1990, results of more than 20 large, *long-term* trials with more than 20000 patients enrolled have given overwhelming evidence that β-blockers reduce overall mortality, reinfarction and sudden death (Yusuf et al. 1985; Frishman 1992; Held 1993; Hampton 1994). In the largest of the *early* intervention trials (>16000 patients studied), mortality was reduced by 15% during the first 7 days of treatment (mortality: 3.9% in the β-blocker group, 4.6% in the control group; $p<0.05$; ISIS-1 1986). When analyzed for separate time intervals, mortality reduction was most extensive during the first 2 days ($\sim25\%$) so that maximum benefit is most likely when treatment is initiated early. Analyses of the causes of death suggest that the reduction of mortality during early β-blocker treatment is mainly due to prevention of cardiac rupture and ventricular fibrillation (ISIS-1 1988).

While in ISIS-1 and other studies only early beneficial effects of β-blockers have been investigated (e.g., for 7 days in the ISIS-1 trial, 1986), in various trials effects of β-blockade on the prevention of myocardial infarction have been evaluated during long-term treatment. Distinguishing studies in which β-blockers were given early (within 24 h of the acute episode) from those in which β-blockers were given late (treatment start 24 h or more days after MI) reflects a clinically relevant decision, although it seems to be arbitrary.

Yusuf et al. (1985) analyzed more than 60 post-infarction trials suggesting that β-blockers reduce death by about 20%–25%. However, the aim of Yusuf et al.'s detailed meta-analysis was to prove if β-blockade in acute myocardial infarction is beneficial at all. It contains no further advice to clinicians on which patient should be treated by which particular β-blocker at which dose and at which stage of the illness. Comparative studies investigating effects of different β-blockers are lacking, so we have to compare different individual trials to answer the questions implied above. Our analysis is restricted to trials involving more than 100 patients per treatment group (see Table 1; one smaller trial investigating the newer β-blocking drug carvedilol is included for comparison).

More than 20 major randomized, controlled trials with β-blockers have been reported, with treatment and mean follow-up ranging from several months to 6 years. Most of these trials have been conducted in the prethrombolytic era. On the basis of multiple, long-term clinical studies, the effectiveness of β-blockers with regard to mortality and morbidity in survivors of an acute myocardial infarction has been proven (Frishman et al. 1984a; Yusuf et al. 1985). In the larger trials, nine different β-blockers were studied with regard to total mortality, cardiovascular mortality, sudden death and nonfatal reinfarction. All of these trials were double-blind and included a placebo control group. Study populations varied from 230 to nearly 4000 patients (Ahlmark and Saetre 1976; Andersen et al. 1979; Australian and Swedish Pindolol Study Group 1983; Baber et al. 1980; Barber et al. 1976; BHAT 1982; Boissel et al. 1990; European Infarction Study Group 1984; Hansteen et al. 1982; Julian et al. 1982; Lopressor Study Group 1987; Norwegian Multicentre Study Group 1981; Taylor et al. 1982; Wilhelmsson et al. 1974). A meta-analysis of these data suggests that the risk of death was reduced from $\sim 9.6\%$ to $\sim 7.7\%$ (chi-square test: $p<0.001$), i.e., an overall risk reduction of $\sim 20\%$.

For statistical reasons, only the larger trials could demonstrate a statistically significant, beneficial effect on total mortality (Fig. 1, larger symbols): in the Norwegian Multicentre Trial (1981) the effects of 10 mg timolol bid on mortality and arrhythmias were studied. Treatment was started between 7 and 28 days after acute myocardial infarction. As for most trials, patients with acute heart failure, hypotension, bradycardia, AV block or obstructive pulmonary disease were excluded. In an intention-to-treat analysis, a significant risk reduction of $\sim 35\%$ ($p = 0.002$) was demonstrated. In the BHAT trial (1982) 1921 patients were randomized to placebo and 1916 patients to propranolol 60–80 mg tds. Patients were included 5–21 days post-MI, and followed for a median of 2 years. Active treatment significantly reduced mortality from 9.8% to 7.2% ($p=0.004$). In the large Multicenter Interna-

chronic beta-blockade in secondary prevention of MI
- results of main trials: mortality -

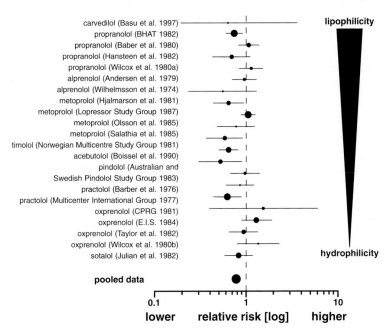

Fig. 1. Mortality data of major clinical trials on chronic *β*-blockade in the secondary prevention of myocardial infarction. *Size of dots* represents the size of study population. The *bars* represent the 95% confidence interval for the change of relative risk due to therapy. Trials are listed in order of the lipophilicity of the drugs investigated

tional Group Study (Multicenter International Group 1977) more than 3000 patients were enrolled to receive either placebo or practolol (200 mg bid). A significant risk reduction by about 38% was observed ($p = 0.007$). Due to serious oculomucocutaneous side effects, practolol is currently not used in clinical practice. Other studies randomizing more than 500 patients each did not demonstrate a significant risk reduction (metoprolol, Lopressor Study Group 1987; propranolol, Hansteen et al. 1982; sotalol, Julian et al. 1982; or pindolol, Australian and Swedish Pindolol Study Group 1983); some studies even demonstrated a trend towards increased risk (oxprenolol; E.I.S 1984, CPRG 1981). Although most *β*-blocker studies testing compounds with intrinsic sympathomimetic activity (ISA) have shown no risk reduction or even a trend towards increased risk in secondary prevention of MI (pindolol, oxprenolol), acebutolol, with its low to moderate ISA, significantly reduced mortality from 11.0% in the placebo group to 5.7% in the group allocated to β-blocker treatment during 1 year of treatment ($p = 0.02$; Boissel et al. 1990). This initial reduction of mortality during acebutolol treatment was even observed in a 5-year follow-up survey (Cucherat et al. 1997), although the controlled trial situation was stopped after 1-year of treatment.

In early-entry, long-term trials, metoprolol (15 mg i.v. followed by 200 mg bid po; Salathia et al. 1985; or followed by 100 mg bid; Hjalmarson et al. 1981) significantly reduced mortality from 11.8% to 6.9% ($p = 0.02$; Salathia et al. 1985) and from 8.9% to 5.7% ($p = 0.02$; Hjalmarson et al. 1981), respectively. Early (within 6 h) intravenous administration of alprenolol (5 mg) followed by a 1-year treatment with 200 mg oral alprenolol per day only slightly reduced overall mortality (risk reduction ∼5%; n.s.). Similar trends were obtained by early oral treatment followed by a chronic oral treatment regimen with practolol (Barber et al. 1976) and propranolol or atenolol (Wilcox 1980a). Treatment with oxprenolol showed a trend towards higher death rates (Wilcox 1980b).

Interesting results have been obtained with randomized short-term studies in which patients were followed for the period past discontinuation of β-blockade: in the ISIS-1 trial (ISIS-1 1986) patients received intravenous atenolol (5–10 mg) followed by oral atenolol (100 mg/day) for 1 week. While there was a significant 15% risk reduction at the end of treatment (1 week after MI), a minor risk reduction (∼10%) was still detectable 1 year later (ISIS-1). Since nearly the same percentage of patients (26% of the previous β-blocker group vs. 35% of the control group; n.s.) was on β-blockade after discontinuation of the double-blind study period, these "late" effects may presumably be attributed to the early intervention. Similiar results were obtained in a study by Hjalmarson et al. (1981): the significant risk reduction observed at the end of the 3-month treatment with metoprolol was still present 2 years later. The benefit, however, leveled off 5 years later (Herlitz et al. 1988).

The data from all *β*-blocker trials indicate that a policy of starting treatment early with intravenous *β*-blockers and then continuing treatment orally is likely to save more lives than utilizing either strategy alone (Yusuf et al. 1988). Early treatment effects seem to still be detectable a few years later, but benefit of treatment probably diminishes gradually over the years until it has disappeared after ~5 years (Herlitz et al. 1988). Although most of the large *β*-blocker trials have been conducted in the prethrombolytic era, results of a recent study with intravenous carvedilol followed by chronic oral treatment nevertheless suggests favorable effects of *β*-blockers in patients with acute myocardial infarction and coronary recanalization by thrombolysis (Basu et al. 1997). Thus, use of *β*-blockers in secondary prevention of myocardial infarction has to be strictly encouraged (ACC/AHA Task Force 1996). The combination of intravenous *β*-blockade and ACE inhibition during acute myocardial infarction should currently be avoided, since synergistic hypotensive effects have to be expected: until now, these interactions have not been sufficiently studied in randomized, placebo-controlled trials.

Combination of *β*-Blockade and Other Drugs in Secondary Prevention of Myocardial Infarction

β-Blockade After Thrombolysis

During the early hours of a heart attack, jeopardized myocardium rapidly deteriorates into irreversibly damaged tissue. Further, the acutely ischemic myocardium is prone to develop life-threatening arrhythmias, and ventricular arrhythmias are thought to be pivotal prognostic factors in postinfarction patients (Kostis 1987). Thus, strategies that reduce infarct size and/or prevent fatal arrhythmias are likely to prolong survival and reduce mortality (Yusuf et al. 1983). The efficacy of early treatment with *β*-blockers in reducing all-cause mortality and ischemic events after acute myocardial infarction (AMI) has been widely accepted, since large clinical trials (e.g., ISIS-I 1986; The MIAMI Trial Research Group 1985) have shown a significant reduction of early mortality by 13% when treatment is started within 24 h of chest pain.

However, most of these clinical trials demonstrating beneficial effects of β-blockers have been conducted in the prethrombolytic era (ISIS-2 1988; Gruppo GISSI-1 1987). Only one large-scale, randomized, controlled trial has tested the effect of intravenous versus oral β-blockade in patients treated with thrombolytic drugs (Roberts et al. 1991). The study failed to demonstrate a significant reduction in mortality by intravenous administration of β-blockade, but did show a reduction in ischemic events. Phase 2 of the TIMI trial (The TIMI Study Group 1989) was primarily designed to investigate the value of early percutaneous transluminal coronary angioplasty (PTCA) after thrombolysis. A subgroup of the patients was assigned to 15 mg intravenous metoprolol immediately followed by oral metoprolol, or to oral metoprolol from day 6. While death rates at day 6 and day 42 were similar in the two groups, there were fewer nonfatal reinfarctions among the patients given intravenous metoprolol (16 vs 31 patients; $p<0.05$) and fewer ischemic episodes (107 vs 147 patients; $p<0.05$).

To date, large trials on thrombolysis do not support the conclusion that effects of thrombolysis and β-blockade are synergistic or at least additive. The ISIS-2 (1988) trial suggests a minor benefit of β-blockade (mortality of 8.4% compared to 9.3% in the group without β-blocker). Another study (Brener et al. 1995), which was also not primarily designed to investigate effects of β-blockade on all-cause mortality, even showed increased adverse events in the group treated with intravenous atenolol.

Furthermore, the negative inotropic effects of β-blockers and their potential to aggravate heart failure have, in most cases, limited their use to patients who did not show signs of heart failure at study entry (Yusuf et al. 1985). However, using the criteria of the BHAT trial (BHAT 1982), some 80% of the patients could be treated with β-blockers, although only $\sim 50\%$ are treated with β-blockers in current practice (Viskin et al. 1995). In addition, a recent study on acute intravenous and subsequent chronic effects of carvedilol on a combined cardiovascular end-point did not show deleterious effects of early intravenous β-blockade. All-cause mortality was reduced, although the difference did not reach significance (Basu et al. 1997). Most patients (>95%) in this study underwent thrombolysis either with streptokinase or tissue plasminogen activator.

Thus, early *β*-blockade may be beneficial even after thrombolysis to secondary prevention in acute myocardial infarction due to its chronic, favorable effects on cardiac remodelling (Mansoor et al. 1996), ventricular arrhythmias (Yusuf et al. 1983), arrhythmic death (Hampton 1994), reinfarction (Yusuf et al. 1988) and sympathovagal balance (Tuininga et al. 1995; Kontopoulos 1996).

β-Blockade and Aspirin

Long-term postinfarction studies of *β*-blockade in coronary artery disease were conducted before the introduction of aspirin into secondary prevention of MI. As shown in the ISIS-2 trial (ISIS-2 1988), the additional use of *β*-blockers appeared to result in a minor additional benefit over aspirin treatment. The fatality rate was reduced by *β*-blockade from 9.5% to 8.0% in patients on aspirin, and from 11.9% to 10.1% in other patients. However, this study was primarily designed to test effects of aspirin, and results with regard to *β*-blockade were obtained in a subgroup analysis. Thus, these results strongly suggest a beneficial, additive effect of *β*-blockers on top of that of aspirin, but do not prove it unequivocally.

β-Blockade and ACE Inhibition

In the early 1990s it was shown for the first time that ACE inhibition significantly reduces cardiac morbidity in patients with chronic heart failure due to ischemic and non-ischemic causes (Pfeffer et al. 1992; SOLVD Investigators 1992). In the meantime, the benefit of ACE inhibition in acute myocardial infarction is well established (ISIS-4 1995; Swedberg et al. 1992), probably due to beneficial effects on cardiac remodelling after myocardial infarction (Konstam 1995; Mansoor et al. 1996). Although it is well known that activation of the neurohumoral system – i.e., increases in plasma levels of norepinephrine – is an established negative prognostic factor with regard to cardiovascular mortality and morbidity (Rouleau et al. 1994), studies with ACE inhibitors have shown that *β*-blockers are still underutilized in postinfarction patients (Rogers et al. 1994; Viskin et al. 1995). The reluctance to treat postinfarction patients with β-blockers is probably due to a common fear of precipitating or aggravating heart failure, although their value is proven particularly in these patients (Gundersen 1983; Yusuf et al. 1985; The Beta-Blocker Pooling Project 1988).

While recent studies have shown the capability of the renin-angiotensin-aldosterone system (RAAS) to influence the adrenergic-receptor expression in a myocardial infarction model (Sanbe and Takeo 1995), there are no prospective studies to investigate potential synergistic or deleterious effects of combined ACE inhibition and β-blockade in the clinical setting.

Vantrimpont et al. (1997) studied this interaction of interventions in the RAAS and adrenergic system retrospectively using data from the SAVE study (Pfeffer et al. 1992). In the SAVE population, the use of β-blockers was significantly associated with lower 1-year and total cardiovascular mortality (risk reduction 42% and 43%).

These and other data (Aronow et al. 1997) give evidence that β-blockade may act synergistically with ACE inhibition. Although drawn on retrospective data, a risk reduction of 35%–40% (Aronow et al. 1997; Vantrimpont et al. 1997) leads to the conclusion that β-blockade may additionally reduce mortality on top of concomitant ACE inhibition. These results are supported by the results of recent prospective trials of beneficial effect of β-blockade in heart failure (both of ischemic and non-ischemic origin), in which over 90% of the patients routinely received ACE inhibition (CIBIS Investigators and Committees 1994; Packer et al. 1996).

These results suggest that combination therapy of ACE inhibitors and β-blockers is safe and may reduce cardiovascular mortality and morbidity synergistically in postinfarction patients, although bias cannot be excluded at this point. Acute β-blockade and acute ACE inhibition in patients with acute myocardial infarction has not been studied, and such treatment should currently be avoided due to the anticipated, synergistic hypotensive effect.

Adverse Reactions, Tolerability and Limitation of β-Blockade

Due to contraindications or side effects, β-blockers cannot be given to all patients with suspected acute myocardial infarction or patients who have suffered myocardial infarction (BHAT 1982). Failure to prescribe β-blockers is common, but reasons are beyond clear contraindications or side effects in most cases (Jansen and Gurwitz 1994; Viskin et al. 1995). Generally accepted contraindications include hypotension (systolic blood pressure <100 mmHg), bradycardia (heart rate of <50 beats per min), acute cardial decompensation, higher degree sinuatrial or atrioventricular block (PQ time >0.24 s), obstructive lung disease requiring medical treatment, Raynauds phenomenon and previous adverse reactions to β-blocking agents (Hjalmarson and Olsson 1991). These contraindications, however, do not explain why in some of the β-blocker studies enrolling more than 200 patients only ∼50% of the eligible patients were included (Frishman et al. 1984b).

β-Blockade is no longer regarded as absolutely contraindicated in patients with chronic heart failure (The Beta-Blocker Pooling Project 1988; Waagstein et al. 1993; CIBIS Investigators and Committees 1994; Viskin and Barron 1996), diabetes (Kjekshus et al. 1990), moderate peripheral vascular disease (BHAT 1982; Olsson et al. 1985) or age (Hansteen et al. 1982; Olsson et al. 1985), although physicians are often reluctant to prescribe β-blockers to such patients (Viskin et al. 1995; Montague et al. 1991). In contrast, β-blockade is especially beneficial in those patients at increased cardiovascular risk (Kjekshus et al. 1990; The Beta-Blocker Pooling Project 1988). Soumerai et al. (1997) demonstrated in a retrospective cohort study that calcium channel blockers are more frequently prescribed in post-MI patients than β-blockers, and underuse of β-blockers, which is of growing concern to both generalists and specialists (Ayanian et al. 1994), significantly contributes to adverse outcomes especially in the elderly (Soumerai et al. 1997).

No significant excess mortality was found in multicenter studies in which β-blockade was started in patients with acute MI but without acute symptoms of heart failure (ISIS-1 1986). In addition, as discussed elsewhere, patients with chronic heart failure may benefit from chronic β-blockade (The Beta-Blocker Pooling Project 1988; CIBIS Investigators and Committees 1994; Packer et al. 1996). To achieve final drug levels in patients with chronic heart failure, drugs have to be titrated cautiously, starting with extremely low doses under close clinical supervision (carvedilol

3.125 mg bid, Packer et al. 1996; metoprolol 5 mg bid, Waagstein et al. 1993; bisoprolol 1.25 mg/day, CIBIS Investigators and Committees 1994 and CIBIS Scientific Committee 1997).

Selection of β-Blockers for the Individual Patient in Secondary Prevention of Myocardial Infarction

The ACC/AHA task force clearly recommends β-blocker treatment for long-term therapy in all survivors of myocardial infarction without a clear contraindication to β-adrenoceptor blocker therapy (Ryan et al. 1996). But which one should be used?

Pharmacological Profile

As mentioned above, it must be emphasized that the widely accepted trials of beneficial effects of β-adrenoceptor antagonists were conducted in the prethrombolytic era: they involved different β-blockers (see Table 1), such as propranolol (with membrane stabilizing activity; BHAT 1982), metoprolol (with β_1-selectivity; Hjalmarson et al. 1981), and timolol (with neither; Norwegian Multicentre Study Group 1981; Pedersen 1985). These agents lack significant intrinsic sympathomimetic activity (ISA), although acebutolol (with low to moderate ISA) clearly demonstrated its efficacy in reducing mortality in post-MI patients (Boissel et al. 1990).

Figure 1 clearly demonstrates that ISA is the only ancillary property of β-blocking that is important for preventing death after myocardial infarction. Propranolol and timolol are both nonselective β-blockers. Acebutolol, which has shown a beneficial effect, is a nonselective blocker with low to moderate intrinsic sympathomimetic activity (ISA; Boissel et al. 1990). Sotalol, a racemate with class III antiarrhythmic activity, did not cause a significant reduction in fatalities, presumably due to the small group studied with low fatality rates in the control group (Julian et al. 1982). Pindolol did not show any beneficial effects (Australian and Swedish Pindolol Study Group 1984). Oxprenolol (with ISA) seems to be the least successful drug among those studied (European Infarction

Study Group 1984); this may be due to its ISA exceeding that of acebutolol. Pure β_1-selectivity (e.g., metoprolol) does not carry any prominent effect (Hjalmarson et al. 1981). To add to the confusion, the drug most obviously successful in the acute intervention trials (<24 h after myocardial infarction) – atenolol – has not been used in late treatment trials (ISIS-1 1986). The only conclusion that can be drawn from this group of trials is that prevention of death after myocardial infarction is probably a class effect common to all *β*-blockers. Intrinsic sympathoadrenergic activity appears to be disadvantageous to treating post-MI patients.

Individual Patient Profile

The *β*-blocker pooling project was initiated to answer questions regarding patient profiles by pooling the data of nine trials involving nearly 14000 patients (The Beta-Blocker Pooling Project 1988). The trials were selected according to the following criteria: (a) randomization within 1–45 days after acute MI; (b) total sample size of at least 200 patients; (c) treatment and follow-up for at least 1 year; (d) double-blind, placebo-controlled trials with mortality data available on an "intention-to-treat" basis. Original data of each trial were included in the analysis. Due to differences in patient selection criteria in the studies, distribution of studied patients in the subgroups analyzed varied. None of the results of subgroup analyses were statistically significant. Thus, conclusions from subgroup analysis have to be drawn with caution.

The key results are the following:

- *Age.* Patients older than 50 years seem to benefit from long-term *β*-blockade. The age group of 50- to 59-years-olds appeared to experience the greatest reduction in mortality ($\sim 37\%$)
- *Gender.* Beneficial effects of *β*-blockers on mortality appear to be comparable in both sexes.
- *Start of Treatment.* Patients seem to benefit most from an early begin of treatment.
- *Prior Cardiovascular Disease.* Patients with prior MI, angina pectoris, hypertension, or treatment with digitalis had an above-average placebo group mortality; in these subgroups there was a marked reduction of mortality by *β*-blocker treatment.

- *Symptoms During MI.* Patients with myocardial failure or with increased heart rate do not appear to benefit very much from β-blockade, while treatment of arterial hypertension by β-blockers seems to be beneficial.

The results of the BBP project must be discussed carefully: high-risk patients were the ones who benefited greatly from active treatment with β-adrenergic receptor antagonist. The major drawback of these calculations is that some studies are more often represented in particular subgroups than others. Thus, ambiguous results may be due to different inclusion and exclusion criteria of the individual studies. Besides this pooling project, subgroup analyses have also been particularly extensive in the timolol trial (Rodda 1983): effects seen in the total sample were also seen in different subgroups. No major subgroups were identified for which a positive effect could be excluded. In addition, detailed analyses of the influence of age (Gundersen et al. 1982) and heart size (Gundersen 1983) showed comparable benefits of therapy in all subgroups examined.

Effects on Heart Rate

Heart rate has been shown to have prognostic importance in acute and long-term follow-up trials after myocardial infarction (Webb et al. 1972; Barber et al., BHAT 1982; Madson et al. 1984; Hjalmarson et al. 1990), as heart rate may reflect deleterious neurohumoral activation (Cohn et al. 1984; Rouleau et al. 1993). β-Blockers reduce resting heart rate (Kjekshus 1986), with the extent of reduction depending on the drug dose and the β-blocker used and on the level of heart rate before treatment. Patients with a sinus rhythm of ≤ 55 beats/min in fact show only a minor effect of β-blockade (Mueller et al. 1974), and in the Göteborg Metoprolol Trial metoprolol did not have any effect on infarct size in patients with low resting heart rates of <70 beats/min before treatment (Herlitz et al. 1984). As demonstrated by Kjekshus (1986), reductions in heart rate differ greatly among clinical trials (from 10.5% to 22.8%). Nevertheless, it is noteworthy that the changes in heart rate correlate with the reduction of infarct size, probably due to a decrease in myocardial oxygen consumption in acute intervention trials. In addition, long-term intervention trials support these hypotheses derived from acute trials with β-blockade: in the trials with larger study populations, significant correlations between heart rate reduction and reduction in mortality and nonfatal reinfarction could be established (Kjekhus 1986). However, due to the major differences among the patient populations studied and the variations of study protocols, large clinical studies must still be carried out to clarify prospectively if a heart rate-guided β-blocker therapy may be useful in treatment of myocardial infarction.

Cost-Effectiveness of Secondary Prevention of Myocardial Infarction

Coronary artery disease (CAD) is the leading cause of death in adults, being responsible for more than one of every four deaths (Kannel and Thom 1994). While stopping smoking, losing weight, engaging in physical activity etc. are easy and inexpensive ways to reduce cardiovascular morbidity and mortality (costs of <$1500 per life year saved; Tengs et al. 1995), medical treatment strategies for prevention of CAD cause huge costs: in 1989, CAD was responsible for about $20 billion in direct medical costs and about $32 billion in indirect economic costs in the United States (Kannel and Thom 1994). Some authors (Frishman et al. 1984b; O'Rourke 1986) even argued against routine use of β-blockers in low-risk patients as costs would outweigh calculated benefit. Yusuf et al. (1988) estimated that β-blockers could reduce mortality by about 20%–25% in secondary prevention of myocardial infarction. Using the main results of these analyses, Goldman et al. (1988) calculated the costs and effectiveness of routine therapy with adrenergic β-receptor antagonists in men. The authors separated patients according to age (45, 55 and 65 years) and cardiovascular prognosis (low-, medium-, and high-risk).

The cost effectiveness of administering β-blockers for the first 6 years after myocardial infarction did not vary substantially for patients of different ages. Using a conservative assumption, about $24000 have to be spent per year of life saved in low-risk patients. Costs are reduced to ~25% in medium- and to ~15% (~$3600) in high-risk patients. Calculated costs do not differ dramatically from these results when in treatment >6 years after MI different models of cardiovascular risk reduction and/or higher costs for drug treatment are added to the analysis. Compared with other cardiologic interventions, such as coronary artery bypass grafting with ~$2600–$100000 per year of life saved, depending on cardiovascular risk (Tengs et al. 1995), or lipid-lowering therapy with $17000–$150000 per life year saved, depending on cardiovascular risk constellation (Hamilton et al. 1995), secondary prevention in myocardial infarction with β-blockers is accepted as relatively cost-effective. In addition, treatment of mild diastolic hypertension (95–104 mmHg) is as cost-effective as β-adrenergic antagonist therapy in the low-risk, post-MI patient (Goldman et al. 1988).

In conclusion, treatment costs of post-MI patients with β-blockers are regarded as relatively low, even with the conservative assumptions made in the study of Goldman et al (1988). One major drawback of this study is the fact that other socioeconomic effects of reduced mortality and/or morbidity are not included and discussed. In addition, analyses calculating costs of a combined, multiple drug therapy (e.g, with β-blockers, ACE inhibitors, anti-aggregatory compounds, diuretics etc.) are lacking.

Future Directions: New Generations of β-Blockers

Almost all drugs considered in large intervention trials for prevention of ischemic stroke and myocardial reinfarction were already available in the early 1980s. More recently, a new generation of β-blockers with additional sites of action has been introduced in the treatment of arterial hypertension and/or chronic heart failure. The most interesting of these are β-blockers with vasodilator capacities, achieved by a variety of mechanisms, such as α_1-adrenergic receptor blockade (e.g., carvedilol), β_2-agonism (e.g., celiprolol, dilevalol, bucindolol), and dilator actions completely independent of adrenergic receptors (e.g., nebivolol). Some of the drugs in this group have been found to exhibit a variety of potentially beneficial activities, such as carvedilol. Carvedilol is a non-cardioselective β-blocker and specific α_1-blocker, which has also been described as an antioxidant and free radical scavenger

(Yue et al. 1992) with antianginal (Rodrigues et al. 1986) and antihypertensive properties (Heber 1987). In addition, carvedilol is a potent inhibitor of vascular smooth muscle cell proliferation (Sung et al. 1993) and is able to reduce infarct size in various animal models of myocardial infarction (Hamburger et al. 1991).

While all these additional properties may provide theoretical reasons for selecting a particular β-blocker, currently available "hard" data of clinical trials with all-cause mortality as primary end-point do not support the choice of these new β-blockaders in favor of older compounds in patients with CAD or after MI. Different properties of the earlier drugs (e.g., membrane stabilization, lipophilicity vs. hydrophilicity, intrinsic sympathomimetic activity, cardioselectivity) lack clinical significance, endorsing a cautious and conservative view of β-blocker therapy in the secondary prevention of myocardial infarction. As example, clinical trials comparing carvedilol (Young 1992), dilevalol (nonselective β-blockade plus vasodilation by β_2-adrenergic receptor agonism; Omvik and Lund-Johansen 1993) or nebivolol (β_1-selective blocker plus direct vasodilator; Ruf et al. 1994) with "old-fashioned" β-blockers such as atenolol did not demonstrate a more favorable antihypertensive effect of the newer compounds. However, one has to keep in mind that during the early 1980s even the beneficial effects of β-blockers in secondary prevention of myocardial infarction were also under discussion. Comparative studies of new and old β-blockers have involved only a few patients (50 patients at most), and minor advantages of particular compounds may have been overlooked. Certainly none of the newer generation β-blockers has been exposed to intensive investigation in very large trials such as characterized the older β-blockers (e.g., propranolol, metoprolol, atenolol, timolol, acebutolol) during the early 1980s and the ACE inhibitors in the late 1980s and early 1990s. A very recent study by Basu et al. (1997) is the first study in which a significant, favorable effect of a new generation β-blocker, carvedilol, has been demonstrated in acute myocardial infarction with regard to combined cardiovascular end-points (see discussion above; Basu et al. 1997; see Fig. 1 and Table 1). These results are promising, however, major impact on clinical practice should be based on results of trials on well-defined, "hard" primary end-points.

Thus, when selecting a β-blocker for routine management of ischemic heart disease, the results of past major clinical trials are still the basis for decision.

Recommended Doses of β-Blockers and Discontinuation of Therapy

In contrast to drug regimens used in clinical trials, much lower doses are often used in general practice (Viskin et al. 1995). To our knowledge no studies have yet been designed to investigate the optimal dose of β-blockers in the treatment of post-MI patients. Thus, more beneficial results may be obtained by changing individual dosage. As no studies are available to answer these questions in detail, the practitioner is encouraged to prescribe doses as used in the larger mortality studies (see Table 1), these having clearly demonstrated beneficial effects. Although beneficial effects of β-blockers appear to be "class effects," only β-blockers for which efficiency has been proven in larger mortality studies, such as practolol (withdrawn due to serious side effects; Multicenter International Group 1977), propranolol (BHAT 1982), timolol (Norwegian Multicentre Study Group 1981), metoprolol (Hjalmarson et al. 1981; Salathia et al. 1985) and acebutolol (Boissel et al. 1990) can be recommended. In general, β-blockers without high ISA should be preferred in cardiovascular therapy.

While beneficial effects of β-blockade in post-MI patients seem to continue to exist over years despite discontinuation of therapy (Hjalmarson et al. 1981; Herlitz et al. 1988; Cucherat et al. 1997), abrupt discontinuation of therapy is correlated with an increased risk of reinfarction and probably death (Alderman et al. 1974; Miller et al. 1975), especially in high-risk patients with coronary artery disease. Discontinuation of therapy a few hours before general or cardiac surgery should be avoided. Post-MI patients seem to benefit from β-blocker treatment during general anesthesia and open heart surgery compared with patients on placebo (Slogoff et al. 1978; Oka et al. 1980); yet clinicians are often reluctant to use β-blockers because of their potential for aggravating heart failure (Viljoen et al. 1972). If discontinuation of β-blocker therapy is necessary due to related side effects, a cautious dose reduction is mandatory for patients with moderate or high cardiovascular risk profile, followed by cessation of therapy after a 1- to 2-week period (Frishman 1987). Even at low risk, β-blocker withdrawal should occur stepwise with complete discontinuation not before 1 week.

Summary and Conclusion

During the past 30 years, various pharmacological and non-pharmacological regimens for the acute treatment and primary and secondary prevention of myocardial infarction have been investigated. In addition to changes in lifestyle, pharmacological interventions comprising antiaggregatory therapies, thrombolysis, ACE inhibition, lipid lowering and β-blockade have proven to be beneficial interventions. Optimal cardioprotective therapy appears to comprise various interventions to achieve maximum efficacy.

Due to infrequent side effects, a high level of safety, and the convincing evidence of reduced mortality, β-blockers have been introduced in the standard treatment of acute myocardial infarction and secondary prevention of coronary artery disease during the past 10 years (Le Feuvre et al. 1996). Unfortunately, this treatment strategy is still underused (Viskin et al. 1995), especially by clinicians without specialty (Jollis et al. 1996). Although most of the studies investigating the efficacy of β-blockade were conducted in the prethrombolytic era and before the introduction of ACE inhibition, combination therapy with β-blockers added has been supported by some recent studies (Roberts et al. 1991; CIBIS Investigators and Committees 1994; Vantrimpont et al. 1997; Basu et al. 1997; Packer et al. 1996). Patients at "higher cardiovascular risks" such as older patients and those with reduced myocardial function and chronic heart failure seem to benefit most from secondary prevention of myocardial infarction (The Beta-Blocker Pooling Project 1988; CIBIS Investigators and Committees 1994; Soumerai et al. 1997). However, β-blockade is also still efficacious in low-risk patients. Calculation of their cost-effectiveness also supports the routine treatment of post-MI patients with β-blockers (Goldman et al.

1988), although these calculations utilized data of prethrombo-lytic studies. Calculations including the costs and effectiveness of combining β-blockers with thrombolysis or ACE inhibition are still lacking. Some newer substances such as β-blockers with intrinsic vasodilatory activity appear to promise additional benefits, especially in patients with acute or chronic heart failure (Waagstein et al. 1993; CIBIS Investigators and Committees 1994; Packer et a l. 1996; Basu et al. 1997).

Only few drugs (e.g., acebutolol, atenolol, metoprolol, propranolol, timolol) have been tested in large trials and have proven their efficacy in secondary prevention of myocardial infarction. Thus, only these substances can be recommended for routine use in secondary prevention of MI, although beneficial β-blocker effects are thought to be class effects, at least for non-ISA compounds.

References

ACC/AHA Task Force (1996) ACC/AHA guidelines for the management of patients with acute myocardial infarction. J Am Coll Cardiol 28:1328–1428

Ahlmark G, Saetre H (1976) Long-term treatment with β-blockers after myocardial infarction. Eur J Clin Pharmacol 10:77–83

Alderman EL, Coltart DJ, Wettach GE, Harrison DC (1974) Coronary artery syndromes after sudden propranolol withdrawal. Ann Intern Med 81:625–628

Andersen MP, Bechsgaard P, Frederiksen J, et al (1979) Effect of alprenolol on mortality among patients with definite or suspected acute myocardial infarction: preliminary results. Lancet 2:865–868

Armstrong A, Duncan B, Oliver MF, et al (1972) Natural history of acute coronary heart attacks: a community study. Br Heart J 34:67–80

Aronow WS, Ahn C, Kronzon I (1997) Effect of propranolol versus no propranolol on total mortality plus nonfatal myocardial infarction in older patients with prior myocardial infarction, congestive heart failure, and left ventricular ejection fraction ≥40% treated with diuretics plus angiotensin-converting enzyme inhibitors. Am J Cardiol 80:207–209

Australian and Swedish Pindolol Study Group (1983) The effect of pindolol on the 2-year mortality after complicated myocardial infarction. Eur Heart J 4:367–375

Ayanian J, Hauptman PJ, Guadagnoli E (1994) Knowledge and practices of generalist and specialist physicians regarding drug therapy for acute myocardial infarction. N Engl J Med 331:1136–1142

Baber NS, Wainwright-Evans D, Howitt C, et al (1980) Multicentre postinfarction trial of propranolol in 40 hospitals in the United Kingdom, Italy and Yugoslavia. Br Heart J 44:96–100.

Balcon R, Jewitt DE, Davies JP, Oram S (1966) A controlled trial of propranolol in acute myocardial infarction. Lancet 2:917–920

Barber JM, Boyle DMC, Chaturvedi NC, Singh BN, Walsh MJ (1976) Practolol in acute myocardial infarction. Acta Med Scand 587(Suppl):213–219

Basu S, Senior R, Raval U, van der Does R, Bruckner T, Lahiri A (1997) Beneficial effects of intravenous and oral carvedilol treatment in acute myocardial infarction. Circulation 96:183–191

Beta-blocker Heart Attack Trial Research Group (BHAT) (1982) A randomized trial of propranolol in patients with acute myocardial infarction: I. Mortality results. JAMA 247:1407–1414

Black JW, Stephenson JS (1962) Pharmacology of a new adrenergic *β*-receptor blocking compound. Lancet 2:311–314

Boissel JP, Leizorovicz A, Picolet H, Picolet H, Peyrieux JC, for the APSI Investigators (1990) Secondary prevention after high-risk acute myocardial infarction with low dose acebutolol. Am J Cardiol 66:251–260

Brener SJ, Cox JL, Pfisterer ME, Armstrong PW, Califf RM, Topol EJ, GUSTO-Investigators (1995) The potential for unexpected hazard of intravenous *β*-blockade for acute myocardial infarction: results from the GUSTO-trial. J Am Coll Cardiol Suppl 5A:901–903

Bronner LL, Kanter DS, Manson JE (1995) Primary prevention of stroke. N Engl J Med 333:1392–1400

Campbell RW, Murray A, Julian DG (1981) Ventricular arrhythmias in first 12 hours of acute myocardial infarction: natural history study. Br Heart J 46:351–357

CIBIS Investigators and Committees (1994) A randomised trial of *β*-blockade in heart failure: the Cardiac Insufficiency Bisoprolol Study (CIBIS). Circulation 90:1765–1773

CIBIS Scientific Committee (1997) Design of the cardiac insufficiency bisoprolol study II (CIBIS II). The CIBIS II Scientific Committee. Fundam Clin Pharmacol 11:138–142

Cohn JW, Levine TB, Olivari MT, et al (1984) Plasma norepinephrine as a guide to prognosis in patients with chronic congestive heart failure. N Engl J Med 311:819–824

Coope J, Warrender TS (1985) Randomized trial of treatment of hypertension in the elderly in primary care. Br Med J 293:1145–1151

Coronary Prevention Research Group (CPRG) (1981) An early intervention secondary prevention study with oxprenolol following myocardial infarction. Eur Heart J 2:389–393

Cucherat M, Boissel JP, Leizorovicz A, for the APSI investigators (1997) Persistent reduction of mortality for five years after one year of acebutolol treatment initiated during acute myocardial infarction. Am J Cardiol 79:587–589

Dahlof B, Lindholm LH, Hansson L, Schersten B, Ekbom T, Wester PO (1991) Morbidity and mortality in the Swedish Trial in Old Patients with Hypertension (STOP-Hypertension). Lancet 338:1281–1285

Dargie HJ, Ford I, Fox KM (1996) Total Ischaemic Burden European Trial (TIBET). Effects of ischaemia and treatment with atenolol, nifedipine SR and their combination on outcome in patients with chronic stable angina. The TIBET Study Group. Eur Heart J 17:104–112

Dhurandhar RW, MacMillan RL, Brown KW (1971) Primary ventricular fibrillation complicating acute myocardial infarction. Am J Cardiol 27:347–351

European Infarction Study (E.I.S) Group (1984) A secondary prevention study with slow release oxprenolol after myocardial infarction: morbidity and mortality. Eur Heart J 5:189–202

European Working Party on High Blood Pressure in the Elderly (1985) Mortality and morbidity results from the European Working Party on High Blood Pressure in the Elderly Trial. Lancet 1:1349–1354

Frishman WH (1987) Beta-adrenergic blocker withdrawal. Am J Cardiol 59:26F–32F

Frishman WH (1992) Beta-adrenergic blockers as cardioprotective agents. Am J Cardiol 70(Suppl I):2–6

Frishman WH, Furberg CD, Friedewalt WT (1984a) β-adrenergic blockade for survivors of acute myocardial infarction. N Engl J Med 310:830–837

Frishman WH, Furberg CD, Friedewalt WT (1984b) The use of β-adrenergic blocking drugs in patients with myocardial infarction. Curr Probl Cardiol 9:1–50

Fuster V, Chesebro JH (1995) Aspirin for primary prevention of coronary disease. Eur Heart J 16(Suppl E):16–20

GISSI-1: Gruppo Italiano per lo Studio della Streptochinasi nell'infarto Miocardico (1987) Long-term effects of intravenous thrombolysis in acute myocardial infarction: final report of the GISSI study. Lancet 2:871–875

Goldman L, Sia STB, Cook EF, Rutherford JD, Weinstein MC (1988) Costs and effectiveness of routine therapy with long-term β-adrenergic antagonists after acute myocardial infarction. N Engl J Med 319:152–157

Grimm RH Jr, Cohen JD, Smith WM, Falvo-Gerard L, Neaton JD and the Multiple Risk Factor Intervention Trial research group (1985) Hypertension management in the Multiple Risk Factor Intervention Trial (MRFIT): six-year intervention results for men in special intervention and usual care groups. Arch Intern Med 145:1191–1199

Gundersen T (1983) Influence of heart size on mortality and reinfarction in patients treated with timolol after myocardial infarction. Br Heart J 50:135–139

Gundersen T, Abrahamsen AM, Kjekshus J, Rønnevik PK, and the Norwegian Multicentre Study Group (1982) Timolol-related reduction in mortality and reinfarction in patients ages 65–75 years surviving acute myocardial infarction. Circulation 66:1179–1184

Hamburger SA, Barone FC, Feuerstein GZ, Ruffolo RR Jr (1991) Carvedilol (Kredex) reduces infarct size in a canine model of acute myocardial infarction. Pharmacology 43:113–120

Hamilton VH, Racicot FE, Zowall H, Coupal L, Grover SA (1995) The cost-effectiveness of HMG-CoA reductase inhibitors to prevent coronary heart disease. JAMA 273:1032–1038

Hampton JR (1994) Choosing the right *β*-blocker. A guide to selection. Drugs 48:549–468

Hansteen V, Moinichen E, Lorentsen E, et al (1982) One years treatment with propranolol after myocardial infarction: preliminary report of Norwegian multicentre trial. Br Med J 284:155–160

Hauf-Zachariou U, Widmann L, Zuelsdorf B, Hennig M, Lang PD (1993) A double-blind comparison of the effects of carvedilol and captopril on serum lipid concentrations in patient with mild to moderate essential hypertension and dylipidaemia. Eur J Clin Pharmacol 45:95–100

Heber ME, Bridgen GS, Caruana MP, Lahiri A, Raftery EB (1987) Carvedilol for systemic hypertension. Am J Cardiol 69:400–405

Held P (1993) Effects of beta blockers on ventricular dysfunction after myocardial infarction: tolerability and survival effects. Am J Cardiol 71:39C–44C

Helgeland A (1980) The Oslo Study – treatment of mild hypertension: a five year controlled drug trial. Am J Med 69:725–732

Herlitz J, Holmberg S, Pennert K, et al. (1984) The Göteborg Metoprolol trial in acute myocardial infarction. Am J Cardiol 53:1D–50D

Herlitz J, Hjalmarson A, Swedberg K, Ryden L, Waagstein F (1988) Effects on mortality during 5 years after early intervention with metoprolol in suspected acute myocardial infarction. Acta Med Scand 223:227–231

Hjalmarson A, Gilpin EA, Kjekshus J, Schieman G, Nicod P, Henning H, Ross J Jr (1990) Influence of heart rate on mortality after acute myocardial infarction. Am J Cardiol 65:547–553

Hjalmarson A, Elmfeldt D, Herlitz J, et al (1981) Effect on mortality of metoprolol in acute myocardial infarction. A double-blind randomised trial. Lancet 2:823–827

Hjalmarson Å, Olsson G (1991) Myocardial infarction. Effects of *β*-blockade. Circulation 84(Suppl. VI): 101–107

Hoffman BB, Lefkowitz RJ (1995) Catecholamines, sympathomimetic drugs and adrenergic receptor antagonists. In Hardman JG, Goodman Gilman A, Limberd LL (eds) Goodman and Gilmans the pharmacological basis of therapeutics, 9th edn, McGraw-Hill, New York, pp 199–248

IPPPSH Collaborative Group (1985) Cardiovascular risk and risk factors in a randomized trial of treatment based on the *β*-blocker oxprenolol: the International Prospective Primary Prevention Study in Hypertension (IPPPH). J Hypertens 3:379–392

ISIS-1: First International Study of Infarct Survival Collaborative Group (1986) Randomised trial of intravenous atenolol among 16027 cases of suspected acute myocardial infarction: ISIS-1. Lancet 2:57–66

ISIS-1: First International Study of Infarct Survival Collaborative Group (1988) Mechanisms for the early mortality reduction produced by β-blockade started early in acute myocardial infarction. Lancet 1:921–923

ISIS-2: Second International Study of Infarct Survival Collaborative Group (1988) Randomised trial of intravenous streptokinase, oral aspirin, both or neither among 17 187 cases of suspected acute myocardial infarction: ISIS-2. Lancet 2:349–360

ISIS-4 (Fourth International Study of Infarct Survival) Collaborative Group (1995) ISIS-4: a randomised factorial trial assessing early oral captopril, oral mononitrate, and intravenous magnesium sulphate in 58 050 patients with suspected acute myocardial infarction. Lancet 345:669–685

Jansen RWMM, Gurwitz JH (1994) Controversies surrounding the use of β-blockers in older patients with cardiovascular disease. Drugs Aging 4:175–183

Joint National Committee (1993) The fifth report of the joint national committee on detection, evaluation, and treatment of high blood pressure. National Institutes of Health. NIH Publication No. 93–1088

Jollis JG, DeLong ER, Peterson ED, Muhlbaier LH, Fortin DF, Califf RM, Mark DB (1996) Outcome of acute myocardial infarction according to the specialty of the admitting physician. N Engl J Med 335:1880–1887

Jonas M, Reicher-Reiss H, Boyko V, Shotan A, Mandelzweig L, Goldbourt U, Behar S (1996) Usefulness of β-blocker therapy in patients with non-insulin-dependent diabetes mellitus and coronary artery disease. Bezafibrate Infarction Prevention (BIP) Study Group. Am J Cardiol 77:1273–1277,

Julian DC, Prescott RJ, Jackson FS, Szekely P (1982) A controlled trial of sotalol for 1 year after myocardial infarction. Lancet I:1142–1147

Kannel WB, Thom TJ (1994) Incidence, prevalence and mortality of cardiovascular diseases. In: Schlant RC, Alexander RW (eds) The heart, 8th edn. McGraw-Hill, New York, pp 184–197

Kennedy HL, Brooks MM, Barker AH, et al (1994) Beta-blocker therapy in the cardiac arrhythmia suppression trial. CAST investigators. Am J Cardiol 74:674–680

Kjekshus JK (1986) Importance of heart rate in determining β-blocker efficacy in acute and long-term acute myocardial infarction intervention trials. Am J Cardiol 57:43F–49F

Kjekshus J, Gilpin E, Cali G, Blackey AR, Henning H, Ross J Jr (1990) Diabetic patients and β-blockers after acute myocardial infarction. Eur Heart J 11:43–50

Konstam MA (1995) Role of angiotensin converting enzyme inhibitors in preventing left ventricular remodelling following myocardial infarction. Eur Heart J 16(Suppl K):42–48

Kontopoulos AG, Athyros VG, Papageorgiou AA, Papadopoulos GV, Avramidis MJ, Boudoulas H (1996) Effect of quinapril or metoprolol on heart rate variability in post-myocardial infarction patients. Am J Cardiol 77:242–246

Kostis JB, Byington R, Friedman LM, Goldstein S, Furberg C (1987) Prognostic significance of ventricular ectopic activity in survivors of acute myocardial infarction. Am Coll Cardiol 10:231–242

Le Feuvre CA, Connolly SJ, Cairns JA, Gent M, Roberts RS (1996) Comparison of mortality from acute myocardial infarction between 1979 and 1992 in a geographically defined stable population. Am J Cardiol 78:1345–1349

Libby P, Maroko PR, Braunwald E (1975) The effect of hypoglycemia on myocardial ischemic injury during acute experimental coronary artery occlusion. Circulation 51:621–626

Lopressor Study Group (1987) The Lopressor Intervention Trial: multicentre study of metoprolol in survivors of acute myocardial infarction. Lopressor Intervention Trial Research Group. Eur Heart J 8:1056–1064

Madson TB, Gilpin E, Henning H, et al (1984) Prediction of late mortality after myocardial infarction from variables measured at different times during hospitalization. Am J Cardiol 53:47–54

Mansoor AM, Honda M, Kuramochi T, Tanaka K, Morioka S, Takabatake T (1996) Effects of ACE inhibition and β-blockade on collagen remodelling in the heart of Bio 14.6 hamsters. Clin Exp Pharmacol Physiol 23:43–49

Maroko PR, Kjekshus JK, Sobel BE, Watanabe T, Covell JW, Ross J Jr, Braunwald E (1971) Factors influencing infarct size following experimental coronary occlusions. Circulation 43:67–82

Maron DJ (1996) Nonlipid primary and secondary prevention strategies for coronary heart disease. Clin Cardiol 19:419–423

Medical Research Council Working Party (1985) MRC trial of treatment of mild hypertension: principal results. Br Med J 291:97–104

Miller RR, Olson HG, Amsterdam EA, Mason DT (1975) Propranolol withdrawal rebound phenomenon. Exacerbation of coronary events after abrupt cessation of oral propranolol therapy. N Engl J Med 293:416–420

Montague TJ, Ikuta RM, Wong RY, Bay KS, Teo KK, Davies NJ (1991) Comparison of risk and patterns of practice in patients older and younger than 70 years with acute myocardial infarction in a two-year period (1987–1989). Am J Cardiol 68:843–847.

MRC Working Party (1992) Medical Research Council trial of treatment of hypertension in older adults: principal results. Br Med J 304:405–416

Mueller HS, Ayres SM, Religa A, Evans R (1974) Propranolol in the treatment of acute myocardial infarction. Circulation 49:1078–1087

Mueller HS, Ayres SM (1980) Propranolol decreases sympathetic nervous activity reflected by plasma catecholamines during evolution in myocardial infarction in man. J Clin Invest 65:338–346

Mueller HS, Ayres SM (1977) The role of propranolol in the treatment of acute myocardial infarction. Prog Cardiovasc Dis 19:405–412

Multicenter International Group (1977) Reduction in mortality after myocardial infarction with long-term β-adrenoceptor blockade. Multicentre internationl study: supplementary report. Br Med J 2:419–421

Multicenter International Study (1975) Improvement in prognosis of myocardial infarction by long-term β-adrenoceptor blockade using practolol. Br Med J 3:735–740

Norwegian Multicentre Study Group (1981) Timolol-induced reduction in mortality and reinfarction in patients surviving acute myocardial infarction. N Engl J Med 304:801–807

Oka Y, Frishman WH, Beker RM, et al (1980) Beta-adrenoceptor blockade and coronary artery surgery. Am Heart J 99:225–269

Olsson G, Rehnqvist N, Sjogren A, Erhardt L, Lundman T (1985) Long-term treatment with metoprolol after myocardial infarction: effect on 3-year mortality and morbidity. Am Coll Cardiol 5:1428–1437

Omvik P, Lund-Johansen P (1993) Long-term hemodynamic effects at rest and during excercise of newer antihypertensive agents and salt restriction in essential hypertension: review of epanolol, doxazosin, amlodipine, felodipine, diltiazem, lisinopril, dilevalol, carvedilol, and ketanserin. Cardiovasc Drugs Ther 7:193–206

Opie LH, Thomas M (1976) Propranolol and experimental myocardial infarction: substrate effects. Postgrad Med J 52(Suppl 4):124–132

O'Rourke RA (1986) Clinical decisions for postmyocardial infarction patients. Mod Concepts Cardiovasc Dis 55:55–60

Packer M, Bristow MR, Cohn NJ, Colucci WS, Fowler MB, Gilbert EM, Shusterman NH, for the U.S. carvedilol heart failure study group (1996) The effect of carvedilol on morbidity and mortality in patients with chronic heart failure. N Engl J Med 334:1349–1355

Page DL, Caulfield JB, Kastor JA, DeSanctis RW, Sanders CA (1971) Myocardial changes associated with cardiogenic shock. N Engl J Med 285:133–137

Pedersen TR (1985) Six-year follow-up of the Norwegian Multicenter Study on timolol after acute myocardial infarction. N Engl J Med 313:1055–1058

Pedersen TR, Kjekshus J, Berg K, et al, for the Scandinavian Simvastatin Survival Study Group (1996) Cholesterol lowering and the use of healthcare resources: results of the Scandinavian Simvastatin Survival Study. Circulation 93:1796–1802

Pedoe HT, Clayton D, Morris JN, Brigden W, McDonald L (1975) Coronary heart attacks in East London. Lancet 2:833–838

Pepine CJ, Geller NL, Knatterud GL, et al (1994) The Asymptomatic Cardiac Ischemia Pilot (ACIP) study: design of a randomized clinical trial, baseline data and implications for a long-term outcome trial. J Am Coll Cardiol 24:1–10

Pfeffer MA, Braunwald E, Moye LA, et al, on behalf of the SAVE Investigators (1992) Effect of captopril on mortality and morbidity in patients with left ventricular dysfunction after myocardial infarction. N Engl J Med 327:669–677

Physician's Health Study Group (1989) Physicians health study: aspirin and primary prevention of coronary heart disease. N Engl J Med 321:1825–1828

Pitt B, Craven P (1970) Effect of propranolol on regional myocardial blood flow in acute ischemia. Cardiovasc Res 4:176–179

Portegies MC, Sijbring P, Gobel EJ, Viersma JW, Lie KI (1994) Efficacy of metoprolol and diltiazem in treating silent myocardial ischemia. Am J Cardiol 74:1095–1098

Propranolol Study Group (1966) Propranolol in acute myocardial infarction. A multicentre trial. Lancet 2:1435–1438

Radvany P, Maroko PR, Braunwald E (1975) Effect of hypoxemia on the extent of myocardial necrosis after experimental coronary occlusion. Am J Cardiol 35:795–800

Reimer KA, Rasmussen MM, Jennings RB (1976) On the nature of protection by propranolol against myocardial necrosis after temporary coronary occlusion in dogs. Am J Cardiol 37:520–527

Rich-Edwards JW, Manson JE, Hennekens CH, Buring JE (1995) The primary prevention of coronary heart disease in women. N Engl J Med 332:1758–1766

Roberts R, Rogers WJ, Mueller HS, et al, for the TIMI-investigators (1991) Immediate versus deferred *β*-blockade following thrombolytic therapy in patients with acute myocardial infarction: results of thrombolysis in myocardial infarction (TIMI) II-b study. Circulation 83:422–437

Rodda BE (1983) The timolol myocardial infarction study: an evaluation of selected variables. Circulation 67(Suppl I):101–106

Rodrigues EA, Lahiri A, Hughes LO, Kholi RS, Whittington JR, Raftery EB (1986) Anti-anginal efficacy of carvedilolm a new beta-blocking drug with vasodilating activity. AM J Cardiol 58:916–921

Rogers WJ, Bowlby LJ, Chandra NC, et al, for the Participants in the National Registry of Myocardial Infarction (1994) Treatment of myocardial infarction in the United States (1990–1993): observations from the National Registry of Myocardial Infarction. Circulation 90:2103–2114

Rossi PR, Yusuf S, Ramsdale D, Furze L, Sleight P (1983) Reduction of ventricular arrhythmias by early intravenous atenolol in suspected acute myocardial infarction. Br Med J 286:506–510

Rouleau JL, de Champlain J, Klein M, et al, for the SAVE-investigators (1993) Activation of neurohumoral systems in postinfarction left ventricular dysfunction. J Am Coll Cardiol 22:390–398

Rouleau JL, Packer M, Moye L, et al, for the SAVE-investigators (1994) Prognostic value of neurohumoral activation in patients with an acute myocardial infarction: effect of captopril. J Am Coll Cardiol 24:583–591

Ruf G, Trenk D, Jahnchen E, Roskamm H (1994) Determination of the antiischemic activity of nebivolol in comparison with atenolol. Int J Cardiol 43:279–285

Ryan TJ, Anderson JL, Antman EM, et al (1996) ACC/AHA Guidelines for the management of patients with acute myocardial infarction. J Am Coll Cardiol 28:1328–1428

Salathia KS, Barber JM, McIlmoyle EL, et al (1985) Very early intervention with metoprolol in suspected acute myocardial infarction. Eur Heart J 6:190–198

Sanbe A, Takeo S (1995) Long-term treatment with angiotensin I-converting enzyme inhibitors attenuates the loss of cardiac β-adrenoceptor responses in rats with chronic heart failure. Circulation 92:2666–2675

SHEP Cooperative Research Group (1991) Prevention of stroke by antihypertensive drug treatment in older persons with isolated systolic hypertension: final results of the Systolic Hypertensives in the Elderly Program (SHEP). JAMA 265:3255–3264

Simonsen S, Kjekshus JK (1978) The effect of free fatty acids on myocardial oxygen consumption during atrial pacing and catecholamine infusion in man. Circulation 58:484–491

Slogoff S, Keats AS, Ott E (1978) Preoperative propranolol therapy and aortocoronary bypass operation. JAMA 240:1487–1490

Snow PJD (1966) Effect of propranolol in myocardial infarction. Lancet 2:551–553

Sobel BE, Bresnahan GF, Shell WE, Yoder RD (1972) Estimation of infarct size in man and its relation to prognosis. Circulation 46:640–648

SOLVD Investigators (1992) Effect of enalapril on mortality and the development of heart failure in asymptomatic patients with reduced left ventricular ejection fraction. N Engl J Med 327:685–691

Soumerai SB, McLaughlin TJ, Spiegelman D, Hertzmark E, Thibault G, Goldman L (1997) Adverse outcomes of underuse of β-blockers in elderly survivors of acute myocardial infarction. JAMA 277:115–121

Statistisches Bundesamt Deutschland (1997) Informationen statistischer Art für einen hochindustrialisierten Staat. Mitteilungen für die Presse. Internet Publikation (http://www.statistik-bund.de/presse/)

Sung CP, Arleth AJ, Ohlstein EH (1993) Carvedilol inhibits vascular smooth muscle cell proliferation. J Cardiovasc Pharmacol 21:221–227

Swedberg K, Held P, Kjekshus J, Rasmussen K, Ryden L, Wedel H (1992) Effects of the early administration of enalapril on mortality in patients with acute myocardial infarction. Results of the Cooperative New Scandinavian Enalapril Survival Study II. N Engl J Med 327:678–684

Taylor SH, Silke B, Ebbutt A, Sutton GC, Prout BJ, Burley DM (1982) A long-term prevention study with oxprenolol in coronary heart disease. N Engl J Med 307:1293–1301

Tengs TO, Adams ME, Pliskin JS, Safran DG, Siegel JE, Weinstein MC, Graham JD (1995) Five-hundred life-saving interventions and their cost-effectiveness. Risk Anal 15:369–390

The Australian therapeutic trial in mild hypertension (1980) Report by the management committee. Lancet 1:1261–1267

The Beta-Blocker Pooling Project (BBPP) Research Group (1988) Subgroup findings from randomized trials in post infarction patients. Eur Heart J 9:8–16

The MIAMI Trial Research Group (1985) Metoprolol in acute myocardial infarction (MIAMI): a randomized placebo controlled international trial. Eur Heart J 6:199–226

The TIMI Study Group (1989) Comparison of invasive and conservative strategies after treatment with intravenous tissue plasminogen activator in acute myocardial infarction: results of thrombolysis in myocardial infarction (TIMI) phase II trial. N Engl J Med 320:618–627

Thompson PL, Fletcher E, Katavatis V (1979) Enzymatic indices of myocardial necrosis: Influence of short- and long-term prognosis after myocardial infarction. Circulation 59:113–119

Tuininga YS, Crijns HJ, Brouwer J, van den Berg MP, Man in't Veld AJ, Mulder G, Lie KI (1995) Evaluation of importance of central effects of atenolol and metoprolol measured by heart rate variability during mental performance tasks, physical exercise, and daily life in stable postinfarct patients. Circulation 92:3415–3423

Vantrimpont P, Rouleau JL, Wun CC, et al, for the SAVE investigators (1997) Additive beneficial effects of *β*-blockers to angiotensin-converting enzyme inhibitors in the survival and ventricular enlargement (SAVE) study. J Am Coll Cardiol 29:229–236

Viljoen JF, Estafanous FG, Kellner GA (1972) Propranolol and cardiac surgery. J Thorac Cardiovasc Surg 64:826–830

Viskin S, Barron HV (1996) Beta blockers prevent cardiac death following a myocardial infarction: so why are so many infarct survivors discharged without beta blockers? Am J Cardiol 78:821–822

Viskin S, Kitzis I, Lev E, et al (1995) Treatment with *β*-adrenergic blocking agents after myocardial infarction: from randomized trials to clinical practice. J Am Coll Cardiol 25:1327–1332

Waagstein F, Bristow MR, Swedberg K, et al (1993) Beneficial effects of metoprolol in idiopathic dilated cardiomyopathy. Metoprolol in Dilated Cardiomyopathy (MDC) Trial Study Group. Lancet 342:1441–1446

Waldenstrom AP, Hjalmarson AC, Thornell L (1979) A possible role of noradrenaline in the development of myocardial infarction: an experimental study in the isolated rat heart. Am Heart J 95:43–51

Webb SW, Adgey AAJ, Pantridge JF (1972) Autonomic disturbance at onset of acute myocardial infusion. Br Med J 3:89–92

Wilcox RG, Roland JM, Banks DC, Hampton JR, Mitchell JR (1980a) Randomised trial comparing propranolol with atenolol in immediate treatment of suspected myocardial infarction. Br Med J 280:885–888

Wilcox RG, Rowley JM, Hampton JR, Mitchell JR, Roland JM, Banks DC (1980b) Randomised placebo-controlled trial comparing oxprenolol with disopyramide phosphate in immediate treatment of suspected myocardial infarction. Lancet 2:765–769

Wilhelmsen L, Berglund G, Elmfeldt D (1987) Beta blockers versus diuretics in hypertensive men: main results from the HAPPHY trial. J Hypertens 5:561–572

Wilhelmsson C, Vedin JA, Wilhelmsen L, Tibblin G, Werko L (1974) Reduction of sudden deaths after myocardial infarction by treatment with alprenolol: preliminary results. Lancet 2:1157–1160

Yoshikawa H, Powell WJ Jr, Bland JH, Lowenstein E (1973) Effect of acute anemia on experimental myocardial ischemia. Am J Cardiol 32:670–678

Young PH, on behalf of the INT-CAR-07 (UK) Study Group (1992) A comparison of carvedilol with atenolol in the treatment of mild-to-moderate essential hypertension. J Cardiovasc Pharmacol 19(Suppl 1):113–120

Yue TL, Cheng HY, Lysko PG, et al (1992) Carvedilol, a new vasodilator and beta adrenoceptor antagonist, is an antioxidant and free radical scavenger. J Pharmacol Exp Ther 263:92–98

Yusuf S, Sleight P, Rossi P, et al (1983) Reduction in infarct size, arrhythmias, chest pain and morbidity by early intravenous beta-blockade in suspected acute myocardial infarction. Circulation 67:32–41

Yusuf S, Peto R, Lewis J, Collins R, Sleight P (1985) Beta blockade during and after myocardial infarction: an overview of the randomized trials. Prog Cardiovasc Dis 27:335–371

Yusuf S, Wittes J, Friedman L (1988) Overview of results of randomized clinical trials in heart disease. I. Treatments following myocardial infarction. JAMA 260:2088–2093

Heart Failure

CHAPTER 8

Molecular Organization of the β-Adrenergic System

Daniel K. Rohrer

Abstract

β-adrenergic receptors (β-ARs) form a critical interface between extracellular and intracellular environments, linking signals generated in the sympathetic nervous system to alterations in cellular function at specific target sites. It is now clear that the ability of β-ARs to alter cellular function is dependent on their close association with a large host of intracellular effectors which are responsible for second messenger generation, receptor trafficking, and receptor desensitization. The β-ARs modulate wide-ranging functions, from cardiac and smooth muscle function to metabolism and behavior, and they are common therapeutic targets: agents acting at these receptors are commonly used to treat ailments ranging from hypertension and heart failure to pre-term labor, glaucoma, and asthma. Advances in our understanding of β-AR function derive from many different approaches, including biochemical, molecular biological, and pharmacological disciplines. By continuing to define in detail the mechanisms of receptor activation, expression patterns, and the downstream effectors of β-AR stimulation, investigators now have a better understanding of β-AR function as well as an expanded range of therapeutic targets.

Receptor Classification and Nomenclature

Pharmacological Classification

The β-AR family is composed of three members, β_1, β_2-, and β_3-AR. These subtypes have been identified using both pharmacological and molecular biological tools, and are prototypical G-protein coupled receptors (GPCRs) since they were some of the first members of this superfamily to be pharmacologically identified and cloned.

Functional distinctions between β_1- and β_2-AR subtypes were made approximately 30 years ago based on differences between the two subtypes in agonist potencies and tissue localization [1, 2]. Norepinephrine was initially observed to have greater potency in the stimulation of cardiac and lipolytic responses (β_1-ARs), while epinephrine and several related congeners were shown to be relatively more selective for bronchodilatory responses and vascular relaxation (β_2-ARs). "Atypical" β-AR functions within adipose tissue and gut were later discovered [3, 4], establishing a new class of β-ARs (β_3-ARs) with relative insensitivity to several well known agonists and antagonists which were not previously thought to have β-AR subtype selectivity.

Table 1 lists several prototypical β-AR agonists and antagonists. Many of these display subtype-selective properties which are frequently used to advantage in the therapeutic setting. However these agents are also particularly useful as investigative tools, aiding in the assignment of β-AR subtype-specific functions and signal transduction pathways. Subtype-specific activation of β-ARs can either be achieved by application of non-selective β-AR agonists (such as isoproterenol) in the presence of selective antagonists, or by the use of agonists selective for a particular subtype. Using such pharmacological approaches, it has been possible to define many subtype-specific functions in vivo. For instance, β_1-

Table 1. A brief list of some representative β-AR agonists and antagonists

Beta adrenergic agonists and antagonists			
	β_1-AR	β_2-AR	β_3-AR
Endogenous Agonist	Norepinephrine	Epinephrine	Norepinephrine
Selective Agonists	Xamoterol T-0509	Zinterol Procaterol	CL 316243 BRL 37344
Selective Antagonists	CGP 20712A Metoprolol	ICI 118551	SR 59230A

AR selective stimulation has profound effects on cardiac function, serving to increase both heart rate and contractility. Most of the effects of β_2-AR stimulation are seen in tissues containing smooth muscle, evidenced by the vasodilatory and bronchodilatory activity of agents activating this subtype. Selective activation of the β_3-AR subtype is found to increase lipolysis and relax intestinal smooth muscle. Accordingly, many of the therapeutic uses of agents acting at β-ARs are applied to these systems: β_1-AR agonists are used for short-term cardiac support while β_1-AR antagonists are used in the treatment of heart failure and hypertension, β_2-AR agonists are frequently used in the treatment of asthma, obstructive airway diseases, and pre-term labor, and β_3-AR agonists are being investigated as potential anti-obesity drugs.

The development of so-called "third generation" β-AR blockers has also had a significant impact on therapeutic use of agents acting at β-ARs, especially in the treatment of heart failure [5–7]. While these agents have multiple pharmacological actions, their effect on β-ARs suggest that their mechanism of action is unique, and these drugs may represent novel tools which will help to reveal new information regarding β-AR pharmacology and mechanism of action. Carvedilol is the prototype of the third generation β-AR antagonists. It is known to exhibit non-selective β-AR antagonist activity, α_1-AR antagonist activity, and is a potent anti-oxidant. In terms of its effects on β-ARs, this drug has the unique feature of possessing little or no intrinsic sympathomimetic activity (ISA), while pharmacologically it behaves as an agonist [8]. In receptor binding assays, one of the features that distinguishes agonists from antagonists is the ability to detect a high affinity state (which is thought to represent receptor plus the GDP-bound form of $G\alpha_s$). Despite its inability to stimulate β-AR function, carvedilol can act like an agonist in such binding assays and recognize this high affinity state. Furthermore, a common feature of antagonist therapy is an increase in receptor number, or supersensitization, while agonists if anything, lead to reductions in receptor number (see Section 1.4.3). The use of neutral β-AR antagonists such as metoprolol in human heart failure is associated with increased β-AR density, while patients treated with carvedilol do not show increased β-AR density [7]. Taken together, the beneficial effects of β-AR blockade without the potentially harmful antagonist-induced increases in β-AR density (and potential supersensitivity) have made this a particularly attractive therapeutic agent as well as a new investigative tool for β-AR pharmacology.

Molecular Biological Classification

The ability to clone and express β-AR genes has had a significant impact on defining pharmacological and functional differences amongst β-AR members. Typically, the cloning of these genes is followed by their exogenous expression in cell lines which are normally null for β-AR expression. In this way, any acquired pharmacological phenotype can be attributed to the expressed receptor. Such expression systems are effective at validating (or invalidating) the subtype-selective nature of pharmacologic agents, and aid in defining the second messenger pathways regulated by the expressed β-AR. There are some limitations to these exogenous expression systems, however. One limitation is that cells which are normally null for β-AR expression may not possess the appropriate machinery to mimic the signaling pathway(s) adopted by β-ARs in vivo. Another is the fact that β-AR expression levels in these exogenous systems frequently exceed normal expression levels, creating the potential to saturate preferred effectors and cross over onto non-preferred effectors.

For the most part, the pharmacological and functional distinctions defined for the three known β-AR subtypes has been borne out by their subsequent cloning and molecular biological characterization. The first β-AR subtype to be cloned was a hamster β_2-AR [9]. The proposed structure of this receptor based on hydropathy analysis and its high sequence homology to bovine rhodopsin (and bacteriorhodopsin) suggested that it contained seven hydrophobic α-helices which alternately spanned the plasma membrane, with an extracellular amino terminus and intracellular carboxyl terminus (see Fig. 1). Cloning of the turkey β_1-AR followed shortly thereafter [10], and it was another three years before the β_3-AR was identified by molecular cloning methods [11]. Human orthologs of these β-ARs have all been subsequently identified and characterized [11–13]. At the amino acid level, these human receptors all share the proposed seven membrane-spanning helical

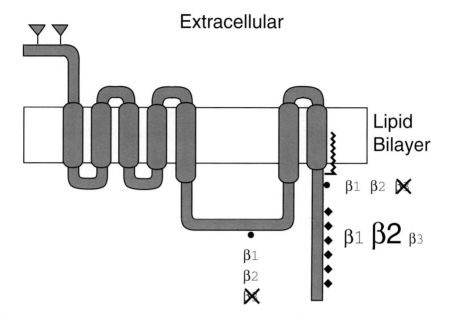

Fig. 1. General topography of β-ARs. This schematic representation of the β-AR is meant to show the proposed basic structure as well as post-translational modifications. N-linked glycosylation sites are found in the β_1-AR (1 site), β_2-AR (2 sites) and β_3-AR (1 site) at the extracellular amino terminal tail. The proposed seven transmembrane segments traverse the lipid bilayer, creating three extracellular and three intracellular loops. The third intracellular loop and proximal portion of the carboxy-terminal tail are involved in receptor-G-protein coupling. PKA phosphorylation sites in the third intracellular loop and carboxy-tail are indicated by circles; β-ARK phosphorylation sites in the carboxy-terminal tail are indicated by diamonds. Crossed out receptors indicate lack of PKA phosphorylation site, while altered lettering size indicates the relative abundance of β-ARK phosphorylation sites in the carboxy-terminus. Palmitoylation site is indicated by jagged line

topology, as well as many other features. Whereas overall sequence similarity at the amino acid level (relative to the β_2-AR) is 54% for the β_1-AR, and 46% for the β_3-AR, the sub-domains of highest conservation reside in the proposed transmembrane-spanning segments. Perhaps not unexpectedly, these conserved helical segments also contain many of the amino acid residues which have been shown to play an important role in the interaction with the catecholamine ligands which bind to these receptors. Notably, Asp-113 of the third transmembrane segment (the β_2-AR subtype will serve as the prototype based on more extensive studies) is thought to serve as the counterion for catecholamine binding: mutagenesis of this residue results in loss of high affinity agonist and antagonist binding [14, 15]. Likewise, Ser-204 and Ser-207 located in the fifth putative transmembrane segment are thought to be important for interaction with hydroxyl groups present on the aromatic ring of several catecholamine ligands [16]. The conclusions which emerge from such structure-function studies suggest that the specific arrangement of transmembrane helices in three-dimensional space form a binding "pocket" for ligands on the extracellular surface [17]. Alterations in receptor structure which result from either spontaneous receptor isomerization or agonist binding are translated to other regions of the receptor, and detected by the myriad host of downstream effectors and regulators, ultimately leading to altered cell function.

The very high relatedness of a given β-subtype across several species (frequently greater than 90% over the length of the receptor in mammals, and even higher within transmembrane segments) suggests that the functional roles of individual β-AR members are well conserved. Pharmacological profiles of either endogenous β-ARs or expression of cloned β-ARs in null cell lines supports this contention: many of the subtype-selective agents developed for individual β-ARs maintain their selectivity across a broad range of host animals, from mouse to man. Table 1 gives some examples of agents which exhibit species conservation of such subtype selectivity.

When comparing different β-ARs, both the intervening loop segments and termini are less well conserved: these regions are thought to be responsible for receptor-effector coupling functions, and contain phosphorylation sites involved in receptor desensitization (Fig. 2). There are clear functional differences between β-ARs in both coupling and desensitization properties, and thus it stands to reason that these divergent regions could play an important part in the subtype-specific differences amongst β-ARs. The largest of the loop regions corresponds to the third intracellular loop

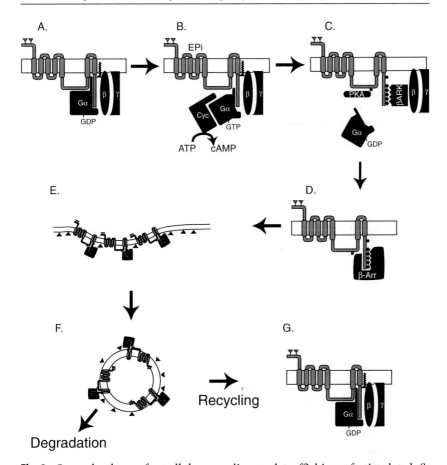

Fig. 2. General scheme for cellular coupling and trafficking of stimulated β-ARs. Membrane-bound β-AR is associated with the inactive GDP-bound form of Gα$_s$, as well as G$_{βγ}$ (A). Upon hormonal stimulation, activated, GTP-bound Gα$_s$ dissociates from the receptor and interacts with effectors such as adenylate cyclase (a membrane-associated enzyme, shown here for convenience as cytosolic) (B). In response to agonist occupation and phosphorylation by PKA (circles) and β-ARK (diamonds)(C), β-ARs become substrates for β-arrestin binding and subsequent uncoupling (D). Cellular microdomains of β-AR clustering where β-arrestin associates with clathrin (triangles) subsequently form (E), and are internalized as coated vesicles (F). Internalized β-ARs can then undergo cellular degradation or recycling (G), after phosphate groups have been removed and receptors returned to the surface. Whereas most of these steps have been established for the β$_2$-AR subtype, details concerning β$_1$- and β$_3$-ARs have not been conclusively established

(between proposed helices 5 and 6), which is 75 residues long in the human β_1-AR. The high degree of structural relatedness between the β-ARs, and indeed between G-protein coupled receptors in general, allows for domain swaps to be carried out between different β-AR and GPCR members. These so-called "chimeric receptors" have helped to reveal many important features of β-AR function. The earliest application of the chimeric technique helped to reveal the role of the third cytoplasmic loop in receptor-G-protein interactions, using an α_2-AR with substitution of the third loop from the β_2-AR [18]. Application of the chimeric technique using different β-AR members has helped to reveal important functional differences between β-AR subtypes as well. Differences in third loop and carboxyl terminal amino acid sequence define important differences in the coupling and desensitization properties of β_1- and β_2-ARs [19, 20]. As well, application of the chimeric technique to compare β_2- and β_3-ARs revealed that domains involved in desensitization are modular and additive [21], while domains involved in receptor sequestration depend on the specific combination of domains, suggesting that a higher order of structure is required for this process [21, 22]. More detailed descriptions of these techniques are found below, *in Receptor Activation Mechanisms and Coupling Behavior*. (Section 1.3).

The ability to engineer such site specific substitutions, deletions or sequence alterations in β-ARs is perhaps one of the most powerful aspects of the application of molecular biology techniques to study GPCRs. These studies make it possible to define functionally important residues and domains, alter pharmacological profiles, and provide a framework for ultimately developing better therapeutics. Another valuable tool contributed by molecular biology is the ability to define the expression patterns of β-ARs in vivo. Whereas in situ ligand autoradiography is a useful tool for defining β-AR subtype distribution [23–27], it is somewhat imprecise in its ability to absolutely discriminate between β-AR subtypes and define expressing cell types. This technique relies on the subtype-specific interaction of radioligands with tissue or cells, followed by autoradiography and microscopic analysis. Some tissue types such as the brain are particularly poor candidates for such analyses, since radiolabelled β-AR antagonists commonly used for this technique such as ^{125}I-cyanopindolol possess

significant cross-reactivity with other GPCRs (e.g. 5-HT receptors). mRNA expression studies and in situ hybridization using labeled nucleic acid probes specific for β-AR subtypes can avoid
some of the pitfalls encountered with ligand autoradiography
since the specificity of interaction is greater, although this technique cannot account for post-transcriptional regulation of receptor
levels. Analysis of mRNA expression patterns has been instructive
for defining β-AR expression patterns in the brain [28], heart [29,
30], adipose tissue [31–33] and lung [34, 35].

The power of combining of pharmacological and molecular biological approaches to the study of β-AR subtypes and functional
analysis is great. However, limitations are inherent to both approaches. Recently, pharmacological evidence has been put forward to support the existence of a fourth β-AR subtype [36]. As
yet, this putative fourth β-AR has not been identified or confirmed by cloning or molecular biological techniques. Moreover,
this new subtype is thought to exist in the heart, an organ which
already has complex β-AR pharmacology due to co-expression of
β_1- and β_2-ARs. Much like the "atypical" β_3-AR, ultimate confir-
mation of such putative β-AR (or GPCR) subtypes awaits identification of a gene product whose pharmacological profile fits with
the observed pharmacology in vivo.

Receptor Activation Mechanisms and Coupling Behavior

The ability of β-ARs to modulate intracellular function is for the
most part dependent on the interaction between activated β-ARs
and the α-subunit of the heterotrimeric G-protein complex [37,
38]. The most common G-protein target is thought to be the stimulatory, a_s-subunit. The so-called "ternary complex model" [39]
was initially useful for explaining the interaction between hormone, receptor and G-protein. This theory stated that the receptor-G-protein complex formed a high affinity state for hormone,
and that upon hormone binding, the G-protein effector could bind
GTP (or related analogs), leading to its dissociation from the receptor. The activated G-protein was then postulated to be free to
interact with its effectors, such as adenylate cyclase. The experimental support for this hypothesis is quite extensive, but recent

experiments have led to slight modifications of this theory [40]. The most obvious of these is the demonstration that receptor activation, previously thought to be regulated solely by hormonal activation, can occur in the absence of agonist or hormone. These results derive from several constitutively active AR mutants [40–42], as well as the demonstration that high level expression of native β_2-ARs can result in constitutive activity [43, 44]. Evidence from other G-protein coupled receptors also supports the notion that basal receptor signaling occurs in the absence of agonist. The "two-state model" [40, 44] can thus account for constitutive isomerization between two discrete active and inactive states of β-ARs (and GPCRs in general). Fluorescently labeled, purified β_2-ARs have recently been used to document ligand-induced conformational changes in β_2-ARs [45, 46], which can also be used to modify interpretations of the two-state model. One interpretation of the results from these experiments is that multiple conformational states are possible, not just two: a series of ligands ranging from partial to full agonists induce a rank order of conformational states which correlate with their ability to stimulate adenylate cyclase activity. Clearly the interactions between ligands, β-ARs, and associated G-proteins is an evolving, dynamic field of study.

In addition to the established role for β-ARs in the activation of α_s-subunits, experimental evidence also suggests that β_2- and β_3-ARs may also regulate signaling through pertussis toxin-sensitive inhibitory $\alpha_{i/o}$-subunits [47–49]. In the study by Xiao, et al., pharmacological data was presented to support an interaction between endogenous myocardial β_2-ARs and $\alpha_{i/o}$-subunits, using pertussis toxin and β_2-AR selective agents [48]. Whereas the existence of myocardial β_3-ARs is still somewhat contentious [31, 49, 50], one study demonstrated that β_3-AR selective stimulation in cardiac myocytes was coupled to inhibitory, pertussis toxin-sensitive responses [49]. The concept which emerges from all of these studies is that β-AR coupling behavior may be somewhat promiscuous and not limited to a single class of Gα-subunit, and that functional responses represent the summation of simultaneous coupling to negative and positive Gα proteins.

The domains of the β-AR which are thought to interact with G-protein effectors (see Fig. 2) have been established by mutagenesis studies, some of which include chimeric receptors. As mentioned above, Kobilka, et al. first demonstrated that a swap of the third intracellular loop region from the β_2-AR into an α_2-AR conferred stimulatory or $G\alpha_s$-coupled responses [18]. Since α_2-ARs normally mediate predominantly $G\alpha_i$-coupled responses, these studies suggested the third loop region was important in G-protein coupling. Refinements of this original observation were subsequently made, implicating the carboxyl terminal portion of the third loop and amino terminal portion of the cytoplasmic tail as playing a role in the G-protein coupling properties of β-ARs [51]. β_1-ARs are known to differ from β_2-ARs by the presence of a proline-rich region found in the third cytoplasmic loop: substitution of this sequence into the β_2-AR reduces its coupling efficiency to adenylate cyclase, while deletion of this sequence from β_1-ARs improves coupling efficiency [19]. Substitution of the seventh transmembrane segment and carboxyl tail of the β_2-AR onto the β_1-AR had no effect on coupling per se, though desensitization patterns were altered [20].

Recent experiments have suggested that β-ARs can also function as dimeric or oligomeric species [52]. By showing that β_2-AR homodimers can be easily detected and that β_2-AR signaling is attenuated when such quaternary structure is perturbed, these studies imply that a new level of signaling complexity is possible among β-ARs, and most likely, GPCRs in general. Whether these higher order structures can be found in vivo, and whether their state of oligomerization can be dynamically regulated remains to be seen, but nonetheless this finding has important implications for dissection of β-AR signaling mechanisms.

The cellular effectors which lie downstream of β-AR-dependent G-protein activation are manifold. The most common and best studied target for β-AR-activated $G\alpha_s$ is adenylate cyclase. Stimulation of this enzyme results in the cellular formation of cyclic adenosine 3'5' monophosphate (cAMP), which in turn is responsible for activation of protein kinase A (PKA). PKA has multiple cellular targets, dependent on the cell or tissue type in question. Activation of this enzyme has pleiotropic effects, ranging from altered gene transcription [53] to enhanced cardiac function. Some of the better characterized targets for PKA in the heart include phospholamban, troponin-I, L-type Ca^{2+} channels, and β-ARs themselves [54–56]. In addition to adenylate cyclase, β-AR-activated $G\alpha_s$ can directly stimulate L-type Ca^{2+} channels [57] or K^+

channels [58]. β-AR-dependent, $G\alpha_s$-*independent* stimulation of Na^+/H^+ exchange [59, 60], has also been reported.

In addition to the targets of β-AR activation identified above, recent experiments have uncovered novel signaling pathways mediated by β-ARs that impact on other, well known signal transduction cascades. Mitogen-activated protein (MAP) kinase activation by the β-ARs [61, 62] has been observed. As well, a significant enhancement of cardiac β-AR function is seen in preparations pretreated with nitric oxide synthase (NOS) inhibitors [63, 64]. In the case of MAP kinase activation, it appears that the $G_{\beta\gamma}$-subunits play an important role in the activation process, whereas the exact interaction between NOS and β-ARs is not well established. In either case, the interplay amongst these different signaling pathways promises to reveal important insights into how different signaling cascades integrate their respective signals to produce the desired effects. Furthermore, a more detailed understanding of the interplay between these multiple pathways will undoubtedly uncover new targets for therapeutic interventions, and further our understanding of signal transduction pathways.

Attenuation of β-AR Signaling

An important feature of β-AR signaling is the attenuation of response which follows repeated or continued stimulation. The molecular targets involved in the attenuation of β-AR signaling include many of the steps in the signaling cascade, from β-ARs themselves to G-proteins. These adaptations which serve to "desensitize" β-AR signaling are implicated in a variety of clinical and pathological settings, in some cases probably playing roles in the disease process itself [29, 65]. Traditionally, β-AR desensitization has been differentiated into two distinct pathways, one termed "heterologous desensitization", the other termed "homologous desensitization". Heterologous desensitization refers to the fact that stimulation of one receptor system, for instance β-ARs, can desensitize responses through *distinct* receptor systems (e.g. dopamine receptors) which modulate the same second messenger pathway. These distinct receptor systems need not be activated in order to be phosphorylated and desensitized. The paradigm established for heterologous desensitization asserts that adenylate cyclase coupled receptors, which modulate cAMP generation and PKA activation, alter function in heterologous receptors by phosphorylation of their consensus PKA phosphorylation sites, whether they are agonist-occupied or not. Homologous desensitization, on the other hand, is thought to regulate only agonist occupied receptors: G-protein coupled receptor kinases (GRKs; also known as βARKs) can recognize agonist bound β-ARs, and initiate a cascade of uncoupling events that start with β-AR phosphorylation (see Fig. 2). Apart from the direct effect that phosphorylation of β-ARs has on coupling behavior, desensitization can also result from receptor sequestration, or removal from the cell surface. In the short term, the sequestration process serves to reduce the density of receptors available to extracellular ligand, and thus reduce signaling capacity. In the longer term, these internalized receptors can either enter a degradative pathway, or be recycled back to the surface. Agonist-dependent changes in β-AR mRNA stability are also known to play a role in long-term attenuation of β-AR signaling.

Phosphorylation Mechanisms

The phenomenon of heterologous desensitization of β-ARs typified by the actions of activated PKA has been appreciated for some time [66]. PKA-mediated phosphorylation of the β_2-AR in vitro results in reduced receptor signaling capacity, with approximately 2 moles of phosphate incorporated (on serines) per mole of receptor [56]. The specific sites involved in this process are found in the third intracellular loop and carboxyl tail [67, 68], although the PKA consensus phosphorylation sites in the carboxyl tail appear to have less impact on desensitization [67]. The primary effect of PKA phosphorylation is to decrease the *sensitivity* of agonist-stimulated β-AR-adenylate cyclase coupling, but not maximal responsiveness [68]. This mode of desensitization can occur at relatively low agonist concentrations.

βARK-mediated desensitization, on the other hand, is characterized by decreased maximal stimulation of adenylate cyclase by agonist, requires higher concentrations of agonist than PKA-mediated phosphorylation, and is specific for agonist-occupied receptors [68, 69]. There are multiple βARK consensus phosphorylation sites found in β_1- and β_2-ARs. The βARK cascade of desensitization begins when agonist-dependent activation of Gα subunits allows βARK to associate with G$_{\beta\gamma}$, followed by phosphorylation of the receptor [70]. βARK phosphorylated receptors can then associate with β-arrestin [71, 72], which functionally precludes further receptor-G-protein interaction. These interactions are schematized in Fig. 2.

Differences have been noted between β-AR subtypes in their susceptibility to desensitization. In general, β_1- and β_2-ARs undergo greater agonist-dependent desensitization than do β_3-ARs; in fact, many studies have shown the β_3-AR to be refractory to agonist promoted desensitization [73–76]. Whereas early evidence argued against the role of βARK in β_1-AR signal attenuation [77], later studies demonstrated a role for this mode of desensitization in β_1-ARs [78, 79]. PKA mediated desensitization of the β_1-AR appears to be qualitatively similar to that found in β_2-ARs [78]. A serine residue present in the third intracellular loop of both β_1- and β_2-ARs is thought to be the primary target for PKA desensitization of β-AR function, which is lacking in the β_3-AR. Phosphorylation sites for βARK reside in the carboxyl tail: there are 10 of these putative sites in the β_1-AR, 11 in the β_2-AR, and only 3 in the β_3-AR.

Other Regulators of Coupling Efficiency

In addition to the well-known effects of agonist stimulation to desensitize β-ARs, the G-proteins they interact with may also be potential targets for desensitization. Cell culture studies analyzing the desensitization properties of both β_2- and β_3-ARs documented reductions in either Gα_s-stimulated adenylate cyclase activity [80], or reduced quantity of immunologically detectable Gα_s [81]. However, in the case of human heart failure which is also associated with reduced β-AR coupling, no evidence for Gα_s reduction could be found [82].

Another potential regulator of β-AR function is phosducin. This molecule is thought to prevent βARK-G$_{\beta\gamma}$ interaction in the unstimulated state [83], though following PKA-mediated phosphorylation (i.e. in response to agonist stimulation) phosducin dissociates, allowing βARK to exert its effects [84]. Whereas addition of phosducin to membrane preparations can inhibit isoproterenol stimulated adenylate cyclase activity [85], the exact role of this protein in modulating β-AR function is unclear at this time. Its widespread tissue distribution suggests it may play an important role in GPCR signaling [85], and its potential to mediate aspects of both heterologous and homologous desensitization pathways is very intriguing.

Dynamic regulation of lipid modified β-ARs may also play a role in coupling state and/or desensitization. The β_2-AR has a well-characterized palmitoylation site at Cys341 which has been implicated in maintaining coupling efficiency for this subtype [86]. More recent experiments have established that the palmitate moiety has a relatively short half-life which is regulated by agonists [87]. Furthermore, PKA-mediated phosphorylation of this subtype is enhanced, and hence receptors uncoupled, in mutants lacking Cys341 [88, 89]. The Cys341 residue found in the β_2-AR is also conserved in β_1- and β_3-AR subtypes.

An interesting observation has recently been made which has important implications for both β-AR desensitization and coupling behavior. Daaka, et al. recently demonstrated that β_2-AR mediated stimulation of the pertussis toxin-sensitive MAP kinase pathway was dependent on the ability of PKA to phosphorylate the receptor [62]. These results imply that agonist stimulation (followed by PKA phosphorylation) serves as a switch, which redirects β_2-AR coupling towards the MAP kinase pathway. If so, our interpretations of what constitutes "desensitization" may need to be modified. These results suggest that what has traditionally been perceived as a desensitization response may actually represent recruitment of a parallel, but distinct coupling pathway with a whole host of distinct downstream targets and effectors.

Signal Attenuation by Receptor Loss

Sequestration and Internalization

In addition to the modifications of β-ARs which influence their coupling function, sequestration or internalization mechanisms which serve to remove β-ARs from the cell surface also have an impact on signaling function. The mechanisms of agonist-dependent internalization have been extensively characterized for the β_2-AR [90–92]. Internalization of the β_2-AR is thought to occur predominantly through an endosomal, clathrin coated pit pathway, although there is evidence to suggest that other pathways for receptor sequestration exist [22, 93, 94], which may differ amongst β-AR subtypes [22]. β_3-ARs are much less prone to agonist-dependent sequestration than either β_1- or β_2-ARs, and the domains involved in this include the second and third intracellular loops as well as carboxyl terminus [21]. Similarly, the β_1-AR is less prone to agonist-dependent internalization than the β_2-AR, and the proline-rich region located in the carboxy portion of the β_1-AR third intracellular loop is an important determinant of this behavior [19]. One important feature of the internalization process besides signal attenuation is the phenomenon of *resensitization*, whereby phosphorylated and uncoupled receptors are de-phosphorylated and sent back out to the plasma membrane [95, 96].

β-Arrestins may serve dual functions in modulating the β-AR signaling pathway: in addition to their effect of blocking receptor-G-protein interactions, β-arrestins are involved in receptor internalization. They appear to function together with βARK to promote β-AR internalization [97], and furthermore appear to be critical for β-AR resensitization [97, 98]. It has also been shown that the clathrin component of these endosomes associates with β-arrestin [99], and that the internalization of such complexes depends on dynamin function [94].

Loss of Receptors

Long-term changes in β-AR density can occur with persistent signaling. Degradative pathways which lead to permanent loss of β-AR density are not well understood, but clearly receptor loss is a common feature of chronic β-AR stimulation, and is seen in many pathological conditions. It is known that long term β-AR agonist stimulation in vivo results in significant β_2-AR loss, with little effect on β_1-AR density [26, 27]. In vitro studies have revealed differences between β_2- and β_3-ARs which suggest that while β_3-AR downregulation is rarely seen, it can occur in some cell types [74]. The carboxyl tail of the β_2-AR is sufficient to impart agonist-dependent downregulation onto the β_3-AR [73]. Human heart failure is also frequently associated with β-AR loss [25, 65, 100], though in seeming contradiction to the above studies, β_1-ARs appear to be selectively downregulated over β_2-ARs in some forms of this disease [101, 102]. The high levels of circulating catecholamines and increased norepinephrine turnover found in many heart failure patients would seem to predict selective loss of β_2-ARs. These results suggest that the complexity of signaling mechanisms which occur in vivo cannot be easily mimicked by common reductionist approaches which tend to study receptors in isolation or out of their proper context.

A recently discovered mechanism implicated in altered β-AR densities is that of mRNA destabilization. It was previously known that β-AR agonist stimulation could shorten β_2-AR half-life, through transcription-independent mechanisms [103]. Studies have shown that the 3' untranslated region of both β_1- and β_2-ARs contain A+U rich regions which can associate with the mRNA binding protein AUF1 [104–106]. Association with this protein confers mRNA instability and eventual degradation, and furthermore, AUF1 is induced by both agonist treatment of cells in culture and in heart failure [106].

New Techniques for Studying β-AR Function

The last several years have seen a dramatic increase in the use of transgenic and gene knockout technologies to better understand β-AR function and mechanism of action. The ability to effect discrete genetic changes in vivo has enabled researchers in the field to expand the range of testable hypotheses, and such studies have had an important impact on the way in which signal transduction is now investigated. Currently, most of these genetic strategies depend on the mouse as a model. The short generation time and ease of housing make these an attractive model system, and furthermore, techniques to study mouse physiology have been rapidly developing, making the whole approach more feasible and pertinent to the human condition. As with any other technique however, there are shortcomings and pitfalls encountered, which must always be considered.

Transgenic Overexpression

Transgenic overexpression of β_1-, β_2-, and β_3-ARs has been achieved in mice. β_1- and β_2-AR overexpression has been targeted specifically to atria [107, 108] and myocardium [43, 109], respectively, while β_3-AR overexpression has been targeted to either brown adipose tissue (BAT) or white plus brown adipose tissue (WAT+BAT) [110].

In the case of atrial β_1-AR overexpression in which the human β_1-AR was fused to atrial natriuretic factor (ANF) promoter sequence, heart rate variability was found to be reduced in vivo [108]. Furthermore, isolated atria from these mice display enhanced basal function, suggesting that constitutive signaling occurs at high expression levels in the absence of agonist. In contrast to transgenic studies performed with β_2-AR overexpressing mice (see below), the functional enhancement in β_1-AR transgenic mice occurs without a corresponding increase in adenylate cyclase function, supporting the idea that β_1- and β_2-ARs have distinct coupling behaviors in vivo.

β_2-AR overexpression has been carried out with human β_2-AR sequences fused to the α-myosin heavy chain promoter, which directs cardiac myocyte-specific expression of the β_2-AR at high levels [43, 109]. Both of these studies document markedly enhanced basal cardiac function, such that the non-selective β-AR agonist isoproterenol has little effect to further stimulate function. As mentioned above, this is associated with increased adenylate cyclase function. The mice created by Milano, et al. [43] were later used to support the two-state model of receptor activation, with the finding that maximal β-AR signaling capacity results from spontaneous receptor activation in the context of high-level expression [44].

β_3-AR overexpression was carried out in either BAT or WAT+BAT in order to define the sites of β_3-AR expression which are relevant to the β_3-AR knockout phenotype. Overexpression of this subtype was performed on the β_3-AR knockout background, in an attempt to compliment β_3-AR deficiencies in vivo [110]. In this series of elegant studies, it was shown that the deficiencies noted in β_3-AR knockouts with respect to insulin regulation, food intake, and oxygen consumption relate to the loss of β_3-ARs from WAT, but not BAT.

Knockout Studies

Genetic ablation, or knockout of β-ARs, has been reported for both β_1- and β_3-AR subtypes [111–113]. Despite the fact that β-ARs are expressed in virtually all organ systems, studies to date have essentially focused on the best known target organs for these receptors. In the case of the β_1-AR, cardiac and hemodynamic function has been assessed [111]. In the case of β_3-ARs, knockout studies have focused on lipid and oxidative metabolism, growth, and endocrine function [110, 112, 113].

Targeted disruption of the β_1-AR in mice is associated with increased prenatal mortality, although the specific cause of death is not known [111]. The penetrance of this phenotype was shown to be strain-dependent, suggesting strain-specific modifiers might play a role in β-AR signaling in vivo. Surviving β_1-AR knockout mice are outwardly normal, although the cardiovascular response to β-AR agonist stimulation is severely blunted: direct chronotropic and inotropic effects of β-AR agonists are completely abolished in these mice, despite the persistent expression of cardiac β_2-ARs. Associated with this functional impairment is a near-complete absence of agonist-induced adenylate cyclase activity. These results were somewhat surprising given the wealth of data suggesting that β_2-AR coupling to adenylate cyclase is more efficient than β_1-AR coupling, both in the heart [102] and in exogenous expression systems [114, 115]. One caveat to the interpretation of such knockout experiments is that many of the previous pharmacological studies were performed with either cloned human β-ARs or human preparations. Unexplained differences can thus result from either fundamental differences between mouse and human β-ARs, or the possibility that previously obtained pharmacological data does not possess the specificity inherent in a genetic knockout.

Targeted disruption of β_3-ARs in mice is associated with mild alterations in body composition, mostly resulting from increased fat content and fat:body weight ratios [112, 113], though this effect is mild in comparison to other genetic models of rodent obesity. The thermogenic properties of brown fat were tested in these knockout mice by cold adaptation, but could reveal no differences between wild types and knockouts [112]. The lipolytic effect of non-selective β-AR agonist stimulation is also comparable in β_3-AR knockouts compared to wild type mice. While failing to show absolute dependence on β_3-AR signaling in the β-AR-mediated control of adipose function, these studies nonetheless validated the pharmacological properties of the highly selective β_3-AR agonist CL316243. This compound has profound effects on several metabolic pathways in wild type mice, but is essentially without effect in β_3-AR knockouts. So even though the effect of β_3-AR loss is mild, the potential for using such β_3-AR-selective agonists as anti-obesity drugs (in terms of safety and efficacy) is validated by this animal model.

While these mouse knockout models can be valuable tools for analyzing receptor function and mechanism of action, our ability to extrapolate from function in mice to that in the human can be problematic. Great care must be taken to show that rodent and human signaling functions are equivalent. One feature of gene targeting which can be exploited in the future is the ability to *replace* mouse genes with those from the human, in essence creating an in vivo reconstitution system. In this way, components of the signaling cascade can be added or removed at will, and tailored to the need of the investigator. The advantages of using a genetically defined system can be joined with the relevance of human genes and gene products. In this way, concerns about pharmacological or structural differences between species can be avoided, and drug screening and testing can much more closely approximate the human condition.

Conclusions

Whereas functional differences between β-ARs have been appreciated for many years, the exact nature of β-AR signaling and the molecular differences between the β-AR subtypes has only recently been clarified. Through the combined use of pharmacology, biochemistry, molecular biology and genetics, the β-AR signaling cascade is being dissected into a number of discrete steps which involve the β-ARs themselves, associated G-proteins, downstream effectors such as adenylate cyclase, as well as the myriad of proteins involved in receptor trafficking, desensitization, and post-translational modification. The continued study of this receptor family will undoubtedly lead to a greater understanding of GPCR function in general, and specifically to better targets and reagents involved in the β-AR signaling cascade. The ultimate goal of these studies is to translate the advances made at a basic science level into therapeutic advances to treat human disease.

References

1. Lands AM, Luduena FP, Buzzo HJ (1967) Differentiation of receptors responsive to isoproterenol. Life Sci 6(21):2241–2249
2. Lands AM, Arnold A, McAuliff JP, Luduena FP, Brown TJ (1967) Differentiation of receptor systems activated by sympathomimetic amines. Nature 214(88):597–598
3. Harms HH, Zaagsma J (1977) Differentiation of beta-adrenoceptors in right atrium, diaphragm and adipose tissue of the rat, using stereoisomers of propranolol, alprenolol, nifenalol and practolol. Life Sci 21(1):123–128
4. Arch JR, Ainsworth AT, Cawthorne MA, Piercy V, Sennitt MV, Thody VE, Wilson C, Wilson S (1984) Atypical beta-adrenoceptor on brown adipocytes as target for anti-obesity drugs. Nature 309(5964):163–165
5. Kendall MJ and Rajman I (1994) A risk-benefit assessment of celiprolol in the treatment of cardiovascular disease. Drug Saf 10(3):220–223
6. Heidenreich PA, Lee TT, Massie BM (1997) Effect of beta-blockade on mortality in patients with heart failure: a meta-analysis of randomized clinical trials. J Am Coll Cardiol 30(1):27–34
7. Gilbert EM, Abraham WT, Olsen S, Hattler B, White M, Mealy P, Larrabee P, Bristow MR (1996) Comparative hemodynamic, left ventricular functional, antiadrenergic effects of chronic treatment with metoprolol versus carvedilol in the failing heart. Circulation 94(11):2817–2825
8. Yoshikawa T, Port JD, Asano K, Chidiak P, Bouvier M, Dutcher D, Roden RL, Minobe W, Tremmel KD, Bristow MR (1996) Cardiac adrenergic receptor effects of carvedilol. Eur Heart J : 8–16
9. Dixon RA, Kobilka BK, Strader DJ, Benovic JL, Dohlman HG, Frielle T, Bolanowski MA, Bennett CD, Rands E, Diehl RE, et al (1986) Cloning of the

gene and cDNA for mammalian beta-adrenergic receptor and homology with rhodopsin. Nature 321(6065):75–79

10. Yarden Y, Rodriguez H, Wong SK, Brandt DR, May DC, Burnier J, Harkins RN, Chen EY, Ramachandran J, Ullrich A, et al (1986) The avian beta-adrenergic receptor: primary structure and membrane topology. Proc Natl Acad Sci U S A 83(18):6795–6799

11. Emorine LJ, Marullo S, Briend SM, Patey G, Tate K, Delavier KC, Strosberg AD (1989) Molecular characterization of the human beta 3-adrenergic receptor. Science 245(4922):1118–1121

12. Frielle T, Collins S, Daniel KW, Caron MG, Lefkowitz RJ, Kobilka BK (1987) Cloning of the cDNA for the human beta 1-adrenergic receptor. Proc Natl Acad Sci U S A 84(22):7920–7924

13. Kobilka BK, Dixon RA, Frielle T, Dohlman HG, Bolanowski MA, Sigal IS, Yang FT, Francke U, Caron MG, Lefkowitz RJ (1987) cDNA for the human beta 2-adrenergic receptor: a protein with multiple membrane–spanning domains and encoded by a gene whose chromosomal location is shared with that of the receptor for platelet-derived growth factor. Proc Natl Acad Sci U S A 84(1):46–50

14. Dixon RA, Sigal IS, Strader CD (1988) Structure-function analysis of the beta-adrenergic receptor. Cold Spring Harb Symp Quant Biol 1(487):487–497

15. Strader CD, Gaffney T, Sugg EE, Candelore MR, Keys R, Patchett AA, Dixon RA (1991) Allele-specific activation of genetically engineered receptors. J Biol Chem 266(1):5–8

16. Strader CD, Candelore MR, Hill WS, Sigal IS, Dixon RA (1989) Identification of two serine residues involved in agonist activation of the beta-adrenergic receptor. J Biol Chem 264(23):13572–13578

17. Strader CD, Fong TM, Graziano MP, Tota MR (1995) The family of G-protein-coupled receptors. Faseb J 9(9):745–754

18. Kobilka BK, Kobilka TS, Daniel K, Regan JW, Caron MG, Lefkowitz RJ (1988) Chimeric alpha 2-, beta 2-adrenergic receptors: delineation of domains involved in effector coupling and ligand binding specificity. Science 240(4857):1310–1316

19. Green SA and Liggett SB (1994) A proline-rich region of the third intracellular loop imparts phenotypic beta 1-versus beta 2-adrenergic receptor coupling and sequestration. J Biol Chem 269(42):26215–26219

20. Rousseau G, Nantel F, Bouvier M (1996) Distinct receptor domains determine subtype-specific coupling and desensitization phenotypes for human beta1- and beta2-adrenergic receptors. Mol Pharmacol 49(4):752–760

21. Jockers R, Da SA, Strosberg AD, Bouvier M, Marullo S (1996) New molecular and structural determinants involved in beta 2-adrenergic receptor desensitization and sequestration. Delineation using chimeric beta 3/beta 2-adrenergic receptors. J Biol Chem 271(16):9355–9362

22. Mostafapour S, Kobilka BK, von Zastrow M (1996) Pharmacological sequestration of a chimeric beta 3/beta 2 adrenergic receptor occurs with-

out a corresponding amount of receptor internalization. Recept Signal Transduct 6(3-4):151–163

23. Rainbow TC, Parsons B, Wolfe BB (1984) Quantitative autoradiography of beta 1- and beta 2-adrenergic receptors in rat brain. Proc Natl Acad Sci U S A 81(5):1585–1589

24. Molenaar P, Canale E, Summers RJ (1987) Autoradiographic localization of beta-1 and beta-2 adrenoceptors in guinea pig atrium and regions of the conducting system. J Pharmacol Exp Ther 241(3):1048–1064

25. Murphree SS and Saffitz JE (1989) Distribution of beta-adrenergic receptors in failing human myocardium. Implications for mechanisms of down-regulation. Circulation 79(6):1214–1225

26. Muntz KH, Zhao M, Miller JC (1994) Downregulation of myocardial beta-adrenergic receptors. Receptor subtype selectivity. Circ Res 74(3):369–375

27. Zhao M and Muntz KH (1993) Differential downregulation of beta 2-adrenergic receptors in tissue compartments of rat heart is not altered by sympathetic denervation. Circ Res 73(5):943–951

28. Nicholas AP, Pieribone VA, Hokfelt T (1993) Cellular localization of messenger RNA for beta-1 and beta-2 adrenergic receptors in rat brain: an in situ hybridization study. Neuroscience 56(4):1023–1039

29. Ungerer M, Bohm M, Elce JS, Erdmann E, Lohse MJ (1993) Altered expression of beta-adrenergic receptor kinase and beta 1-adrenergic receptors in the failing human heart [see comments]. Circulation 87(2):454–463

30. Sylven C, Mischa G, Jansson E, Sotonyi P, Fu LX, Waagstein F, Bronnegard M (1995) Beta 1 and beta 2 adrenoceptor ligand and mRNA expression in dilated cardiomyopathy. Biol Pharm Bull 18(10):1430–1434

31. Krief S, Lonnqvist F, Raimbault S, Baude B, Van SA, Arner P, Strosberg AD, Ricquier D, Emorine LJ (1993) Tissue distribution of beta 3-adrenergic receptor mRNA in man. J Clin Invest 91(1):344–349

32. Collins S, Daniel KW, Rohlfs EM, Ramkumar V, Taylor IL, Gettys TW (1994) Impaired expression and functional activity of the beta 3- and beta 1-adrenergic receptors in adipose tissue of congenitally obese (C57BL/6J ob/ob) mice. Mol Endocrinol 8(4):518–527

33. Evans BA, Papaioannou M, Bonazzi VR, Summers RJ (1996) Expression of beta 3-adrenoceptor mRNA in rat tissues. Br J Pharmacol 117(1):210–216

34. Nishikawa M, Mak JC, Shirasaki H, Harding SE, Barnes PJ (1994) Long-term exposure to norepinephrine results in down-regulation and reduced mRNA expression of pulmonary beta-adrenergic receptors in guinea pigs. Am J Respir Cell Mol Biol 10(1):91–99

35. Mak JC, Nishikawa M, Haddad EB, Kwon OJ, Hirst SJ, Twort CH, Barnes PJ (1996) Localisation and expression of beta-adrenoceptor subtype mRNAs in human lung. Eur J Pharmacol 302(1–3):215–221

36. Kaumann AJ (1997) Four beta-adrenoceptor subtypes in the mammalian heart. Trends Pharmacol Sci 18(3):70–76

37. Limbird LE, Gill DM, Lefkowitz RJ (1980) Agonist-promoted coupling of the beta-adrenergic receptor with the guanine nucleotide regulatory pro-

tein of the adenylate cyclase system. Proc Natl Acad Sci U S A 77(2):775–779

38. Gilman AG (1987) G proteins: transducers of receptor-generated signals. Annu Rev Biochem 56(615):615–649

39. De Lean A, Stadel JM, Lefkowitz RJ (1980) A ternary complex model explains the agonist-specific binding properties of the adenylate cyclase-coupled beta-adrenergic receptor. J Biol Chem 255(15):7108–7117

40. Samama P, Cotecchia S, Costa T, Lefkowitz RJ (1993) A mutation-induced activated state of the beta 2-adrenergic receptor. Extending the ternary complex model. J Biol Chem 268(7):4625–4636

41. Allen LF, Lefkowitz RJ, Caron MG, Cotecchia S (1991) G-protein-coupled receptor genes as protooncogenes: constitutively activating mutation of the alpha 1B-adrenergic receptor enhances mitogenesis and tumorigenicity. Proc Natl Acad Sci U S A 88(24):11354–11358

42. Ren Q, Kurose H, Lefkowitz RJ, Cotecchia S (1993) Constitutively active mutants of the alpha 2-adrenergic receptor [published erratum appears in J Biol Chem 1994 Jan 14;269(2):1566]. J Biol Chem 268(22):16483–16487

43. Milano CA, Allen LF, Rockman HA, Dolber PC, McMinn TR, Chien KR, Johnson TD, Bond RA, Lefkowitz RJ (1994) Enhanced myocardial function in transgenic mice overexpressing the beta 2-adrenergic receptor [see comments]. Science 264(5158):582–586

44. Bond RA, Leff P, Johnson TD, Milano CA, Rockman HA, McMinn TR, Apparsundaram S, Hyek MF, Kenakin TP, Allen LF, et al (1995) Physiological effects of inverse agonists in transgenic mice with myocardial overexpression of the beta 2-adrenoceptor [see comments]. Nature 374(6519):272–276

45. Gether U, Lin S, Kobilka BK (1995) Fluorescent labeling of purified beta 2 adrenergic receptor. Evidence for ligand-specific conformational changes. J Biol Chem 270(47):28268–28275

46. Gether U, Ballesteros JA, Seifert R, Sanders BE, Weinstein H, Kobilka BK (1997) Structural instability of a constitutively active G protein-coupled receptor. Agonist-independent activation due to conformational flexibility. J Biol Chem 272(5):2587–2590

47. Abramson SN, Martin MW, Hughes AR, Harden TK, Neve KA, Barrett DA, Molinoff PB (1988) Interaction of beta-adrenergic receptors with the inhibitory guanine nucleotide-binding protein of adenylate cyclase in membranes prepared from cyc- S49 lymphoma cells. Biochem Pharmacol 37(22):4289–4297

48. Xiao RP, Ji X, Lakatta EG (1995) Functional coupling of the beta 2-adrenoceptor to a pertussis toxin-sensitive G protein in cardiac myocytes. Mol Pharmacol 47(2):322–329

49. Gauthier C, Tavernier G, Charpentier F, Langin D, Le MH (1996) Functional beta3-adrenoceptor in the human heart [see comments]. J Clin Invest 98(2):556–562

50. Berkowitz DE, Nardone NA, Smiley RM, Price DT, Kreutter DK, Fremeau RT, Schwinn DA (1995) Distribution of beta 3-adrenoceptor mRNA in human tissues. Eur J Pharmacol 289(2):223–228

51. O'Dowd BF, Hnatowich M, Regan JW, Leader WM, Caron MG, Lefkowitz RJ (1988) Site-directed mutagenesis of the cytoplasmic domains of the human beta 2-adrenergic receptor. Localization of regions involved in G protein-receptor coupling. J Biol Chem 263(31):15985–15992

52. Hebert TE, Moffett S, Morello JP, Loisel TP, Bichet DG, Barret C, Bouvier M (1996) A peptide derived from a beta2-adrenergic receptor transmembrane domain inhibits both receptor dimerization and activation. J Biol Chem 271(27):16384–16392

53. Lee KA and Masson N (1993) Transcriptional regulation by CREB and its relatives. Biochim Biophys Acta 1174(3):221–233

54. Sulakhe PV and Vo XT (1995) Regulation of phospholamban and troponin-I phosphorylation in the intact rat cardiomyocytes by adrenergic and cholinergic stimuli: roles of cyclic nucleotides, calcium, protein kinases and phosphatases and depolarization. Mol Cell Biochem 150(103):103–126

55. Haase H, Bartel S, Karczewski P, Morano I, Krause EG (1996) In-vivo phosphorylation of the cardiac L-type calcium channel beta-subunit in response to catecholamines. Mol Cell Biochem 164(99):99–106

56. Benovic JL, Pike LJ, Cerione RA, Staniszewski C, Yoshimasa T, Codina J, Caron MG, Lefkowitz RJ (1985) Phosphorylation of the mammalian beta-adrenergic receptor by cyclic AMP-dependent protein kinase. Regulation of the rate of receptor phosphorylation and dephosphorylation by agonist occupancy and effects on coupling of the receptor to the stimulatory guanine nucleotide regulatory protein. J Biol Chem 260(11):7094–7101

57. Brown AM, Birnbaumer L (1988) Direct G protein gating of ion channels. Am J Physiol : H401–410

58. Kume H, Hall IP, Washabau RJ, Takagi K, Kotlikoff MI (1994) Beta-adrenergic agonists regulate KCa channels in airway smooth muscle by cAMP-dependent and -independent mechanisms. J Clin Invest 93(1):371–379

59. Barber DL and Ganz MB (1992) Guanine nucleotides regulate beta-adrenergic activation of Na-H exchange independently of receptor coupling to Gs. J Biol Chem 267(29):20607–20612

60. Barber DL, Ganz MB, Bongiorno PB, Strader CD (1992) Mutant constructs of the beta-adrenergic receptor that are uncoupled from adenylyl cyclase retain functional activation of Na-H exchange. Mol Pharmacol 41(6):1056–1060

61. Crespo P, Cachero TG, Xu N, Gutkind JS (1995) Dual effect of beta-adrenergic receptors on mitogen-activated protein kinase. Evidence for a beta gamma-dependent activation and a G alpha s-cAMP-mediated inhibition. J Biol Chem 270(42):25259–25265

62. Daaka Y, Luttrell LM, Lefkowitz RJ (1997) Switching of the coupling of the Beta-2 adrenergic receptor to different G-proteins by protein kinase A. Nature 390:88–91

63. Belhassen L, Kelly RA, Smith TW, Balligand JL (1996) Nitric oxide synthase (NOS3) and contractile responsiveness to adrenergic and cholinergic agonists in the heart. Regulation of NOS3 transcription in vitro and in vivo by cyclic adenosine monophosphate in rat cardiac myocytes. J Clin Invest 97(8):1908–1915

64. Keaney JJ, Hare JM, Balligand JL, Loscalzo J, Smith TW, Colucci WS (1996) Inhibition of nitric oxide synthase augments myocardial contractile responses to beta-adrenergic stimulation. Am J Physiol, H2646–2652

65. Bohm M, Lohse MJ (1994) Quantification of beta-adrenoceptors and beta-adrenoceptor kinase on protein and mRNA levels in heart failure. Eur Heart J : 30–34

66. Lefkowitz RJ, Wessels MR, Stadel JM (1980) Hormones, receptors, cyclic AMP: their role in target cell refractoriness. Curr Top Cell Regul 17(205):205–230

67. Clark RB, Friedman J, Dixon RA, Strader CD (1989) Identification of a specific site required for rapid heterologous desensitization of the beta-adrenergic receptor by cAMP-dependent protein kinase. Mol Pharmacol 36(3):343–348

68. Hausdorff WP, Bouvier M, O'Dowd BF, Irons GP, Caron MG, Lefkowitz RJ (1989) Phosphorylation sites on two domains of the beta 2-adrenergic receptor are involved in distinct pathways of receptor desensitization. J Biol Chem 264(21):12657–12665

69. Benovic JL, Strasser RH, Caron MG, Lefkowitz RJ (1986) Beta-adrenergic receptor kinase: identification of a novel protein kinase that phosphorylates the agonist-occupied form of the receptor. Proc Natl Acad Sci U S A 83(9):2797–2801

70. Pitcher JA, Inglese J, Higgins JB, Arriza JL, Casey PJ, Kim C, Benovic JL, Kwatra MM, Caron MG, Lefkowitz RJ (1992) Role of beta gamma subunits of G proteins in targeting the beta-adrenergic receptor kinase to membrane-bound receptors. Science 257(5074):1264–1267

71. Lohse MJ, Benovic JL, Codina J, Caron MG, Lefkowitz RJ (1990) beta-Arrestin: a protein that regulates beta-adrenergic receptor function. Science 248(4962):1547–1550

72. Attramadal H, Arriza JL, Aoki C, Dawson TM, Codina J, Kwatra MM, Snyder SH, Caron MG, Lefkowitz RJ (1992) Beta-arrestin2, a novel member of the arrestin/beta-arrestin gene family. J Biol Chem 267(25):17882–17890

73. Liggett SB, Freedman NJ, Schwinn DA, Lefkowitz RJ (1993) Structural basis for receptor subtype-specific regulation revealed by a chimeric beta 3/beta 2-adrenergic receptor. Proc Natl Acad Sci U S A 90(8):3665–3669

74. Nantel F, Bonin H, Emorine LJ, Zilberfarb V, Strosberg AD, Bouvier M, Marullo S (1993) The human beta 3-adrenergic receptor is resistant to

short term agonist-promoted desensitization. Mol Pharmacol 43(4):548–555

75. Carpene C, Galitzky J, Collon P, Esclapez F, Dauzats M, Lafontan M (1993) Desensitization of beta-1 and beta-2, but not beta-3, adrenoceptor-mediated lipolytic responses of adipocytes after long-term norepinephrine infusion. J Pharmacol Exp Ther 265(1):237–247

76. Curran PK, Fishman PH (1996) Endogenous beta 3- but not beta 1-adrenergic receptors are resistant to agonist-mediated regulation in human SK-N-MC neurotumor cells. Cell Signal 8(5):355–364

77. Zhou XM, Fishman PH (1991) Desensitization of the human beta 1-adrenergic receptor. Involvement of the cyclic AMP-dependent but not a receptor-specific protein kinase. J Biol Chem 266(12):7462–7468

78. Freedman NJ, Liggett SB, Drachman DE, Pei G, Caron MG, Lefkowitz RJ (1995) Phosphorylation and desensitization of the human beta 1-adrenergic receptor. Involvement of G protein-coupled receptor kinases and cAMP-dependent protein kinase. J Biol Chem 270(30):17953–17961

79. Zhou XM, Pak M, Wang Z, Fishman PH (1995) Differences in desensitization between human beta 1- and beta 2-adrenergic receptors stably expressed in transfected hamster cells. Cell Signal 7(3):207–217

80. Sibley DR, Daniel K, Strader CD, Lefkowitz RJ (1987) Phosphorylation of the beta-adrenergic receptor in intact cells: relationship to heterologous and homologous mechanisms of adenylate cyclase desensitization. Arch Biochem Biophys 258(1):24–32

81. Chambers J, Park J, Cronk D, Chapman C, Kennedy FR, Wilson S, Milligan G (1994) Beta 3-adrenoceptor agonist-induced down-regulation of Gs alpha and functional desensitization in a Chinese hamster ovary cell line expressing a beta 3-adrenoceptor refractory to down-regulation. Biochem J :973–978

82. Feldman AM, Cates AE, Veazey WB, Hershberger RE, Bristow MR, Baughman KL, Baumgartner WA, Van DC (1988) Increase of the 40,000-mol wt pertussis toxin substrate (G protein) in the failing human heart. J Clin Invest 82(1):189–197

83. Bauer PH, Muller S, Puzicha M, Pippig S, Obermaier B, Helmreich EJ, Lohse MJ (1992) Phosducin is a protein kinase A-regulated G-protein regulator. Nature 358(6381):73–76

84. Hekman M, Bauer PH, Sohlemann P, Lohse MJ (1994) Phosducin inhibits receptor phosphorylation by the beta-adrenergic receptor kinase in a PKA-regulated manner. Febs Lett 343(2):120–124

85. Danner S, Lohse MJ (1996) Phosducin is a ubiquitous G-protein regulator. Proc Natl Acad Sci U S A 93(19):10145–10150

86. O'Dowd BF, Hnatowich M, Caron MG, Lefkowitz RJ, Bouvier M (1989) Palmitoylation of the human beta 2-adrenergic receptor. Mutation of Cys341 in the carboxyl tail leads to an uncoupled nonpalmitoylated form of the receptor. J Biol Chem 264(13):7564–7569

87. Loisel TP, Adam L, Hebert TE, Bouvier M (1996) Agonist stimulation increases the turnover rate of beta 2AR-bound palmitate and promotes receptor depalmitoylation. Biochemistry 35(49):15923–15932
88. Moffett S, Mouillac B, Bonin H, Bouvier M (1993) Altered phosphorylation and desensitization patterns of a human beta 2-adrenergic receptor lacking the palmitoylated Cys341. Embo J 12(1):349–356
89. Moffett S, Adam L, Bonin H, Loisel TP, Bouvier M, Mouillac B (1996) Palmitoylated cysteine 341 modulates phosphorylation of the beta2-adre-
nergic receptor by the cAMP-dependent protein kinase. J Biol Chem 271(35):21490–21497
90. von Zastrow M, Kobilka BK (1992) Ligand-regulated internalization and recycling of human beta 2-adrenergic receptors between the plasma membrane and endosomes containing transferrin receptors. J Biol Chem 267(5):3530–3538
91. von Zastrow M, Link R, Daunt D, Barsh G, Kobilka B (1993) Subtype-specific differences in the intracellular sorting of G protein-coupled receptors. J Biol Chem 268(2):763–766
92. von Zastrow M, Kobilka BK (1994) Antagonist-dependent and -independent steps in the mechanism of adrenergic receptor internalization. J Biol Chem 269(28):18448–18552
93. Strader CD, Sibley DR, Lefkowitz RJ (1984) Association of sequestered beta-adrenergic receptors with the plasma membrane: a novel mechanism for receptor down regulation. Life Sci 35(15):1601–1610
94. Zhang J, Ferguson S, Barak LS, Menard L, Caron MG (1996) Dynamin and beta-arrestin reveal distinct mechanisms for G protein-coupled receptor internalization. J Biol Chem 271(31):18302–18305
95. Yu SS, Lefkowitz RJ, Hausdorff WP (1993) Beta-adrenergic receptor sequestration. A potential mechanism of receptor resensitization. J Biol Chem 268(1):337–341
96. Krueger KM, Daaka Y, Pitcher JA, Lefkowitz RJ (1997) The role of sequestration in G protein-coupled receptor resensitization. Regulation of beta2-adrenergic receptor dephosphorylation by vesicular acidification. J Biol Chem 272(1):5–8
97. Ferguson SS, Downey WR, Colapietro AM, Barak LS, Menard L, Caron MG (1996) Role of beta-arrestin in mediating agonist-promoted G protein-coupled receptor internalization. Science 271(5247):363–366
98. Zhang J, Barak LS, Winkler KE, Caron MG, Ferguson SG (1997) A central role for Beta-arrestins and clathrin-coated vesicle-mediated endocytosis in Beta-2 adrenergic receptor resensitization. J Biol Chem 272(43):27005–27014
99. Goodman OJ, Krupnick JG, Santini F, Gurevich VV, Penn RB, Gagnon AW, Keen JH, Benovic JL (1996) Beta-arrestin acts as a clathrin adaptor in endocytosis of the beta2-adrenergic receptor. Nature 383(6599):447–450
100. Bristow MR, Ginsburg R, Minobe W, Cubicciotti RS, Sageman WS, Lurie K, Billingham ME, Harrison DC, Stinson EB (1982) Decreased cate-

cholamine sensitivity and beta-adrenergic-receptor density in failing human hearts. N Engl J Med 307(4):205–211

101. Bristow MR, Ginsburg R, Umans V, Fowler M, Minobe W, Rasmussen R, Zera P, Menlove R, Shah P, Jamieson S, et al (1986) Beta 1- and beta 2-adrenergic-receptor subpopulations in nonfailing and failing human ventricular myocardium: coupling of both receptor subtypes to muscle contraction and selective beta 1-receptor down-regulation in heart failure. Circ Res 59(3):297–309

102. Brodde OE (1991) Beta 1- and beta 2-adrenoceptors in the human heart: properties, function, alterations in chronic heart failure [published erratum appears in Pharmacol Rev 1991 Sep; 43(3):350]. Pharmacol Rev 43(2):203–242

103. Hadcock JR, Wang HY, Malbon CC (1989) Agonist-induced destabilization of beta-adrenergic receptor mRNA. Attenuation of glucocorticoid-induced up-regulation of beta-adrenergic receptors. J Biol Chem 264(33):19928–19933

104. Port JD, Huang LY, Malbon CC (1992) Beta-adrenergic agonists that down-regulate receptor mRNA up-regulate a M(r) 35,000 protein(s) that selectively binds to beta-adrenergic receptor mRNAs. J Biol Chem 267(33):24103–24108

105. Huang LY, Tholanikunnel BG, Vakalopoulou E, Malbon CC (1993) The M(r) 35,000 beta-adrenergic receptor mRNA-binding protein induced by agonists requires both an AUUUA pentamer and U-rich domains for RNA recognition. J Biol Chem 268(34):25769–25775

106. Pende A, Tremmel KD, DeMaria CT, Blaxall BC, Minobe WA, Sherman JA, Bisognano JD, Bristow MR, Brewer G, Port J (1996) Regulation of the mRNA-binding protein AUF1 by activation of the beta-adrenergic receptor signal transduction pathway. J Biol Chem 271(14):8493–8501

107. Bertin B, Mansier P, Makeh I, Briand P, Rostene W, Swynghedauw B, Strosberg AD (1993) Specific atrial overexpression of G protein coupled human beta 1 adrenoceptors in transgenic mice. Cardiovasc Res 27(9):1606–1612

108. Mansier P, Medigue C, Charlotte N, Vermeiren C, Coraboeuf E, Deroubai E, Ratner E, Chevalier B, Clairambault J, Carre F, Dahkli T, Bertin B, Briand P, Strosberg D, Swynghedauw B (1996) Decreased heart rate variability in transgenic mice overexpressing atrial beta 1-adrenoceptors. Am J Physiol : H1465–1472

109. Turki J, Lorenz JN, Green SA, Donnelly ET, Jacinto M, Liggett SB (1996) Myocardial signaling defects and impaired cardiac function of a human beta 2-adrenergic receptor polymorphism expressed in transgenic mice. Proc Natl Acad Sci U S A 93(19):10483–10488

110. Grujic D, Susulic VS, Harper ME, Himms HJ, Cunningham BA, Corkey BE, Lowell BB (1997) Beta3-adrenergic receptors on white and brown adipocytes mediate beta3-selective agonist-induced effects on energy expenditure, insulin secretion, food intake. A study using transgenic and gene knockout mice. J Biol Chem 272(28):17686–17693

111. Rohrer DK, Desai KH, Jasper JR, Stevens ME, Regula DJ, Barsh GS, Bernstein D, Kobilka BK (1996) Targeted disruption of the mouse beta1-adrenergic receptor gene: developmental and cardiovascular effects. Proc Natl Acad Sci U S A 93(14):7375–7380

112. Susulic VS, Frederich RC, Lawitts J, Tozzo E, Kahn BB, Harper ME, Himms HJ, Flier JS, Lowell BB (1995) Targeted disruption of the beta 3-adrenergic receptor gene. J Biol Chem 270(49):29483–29492

113. Revelli JP, Preitner F, Samec S, Muniesa P, Kuehne F, Boss O, Vassalli JD, Dulloo A, Seydoux J, Giacobino JP, Huarte J, Ody C (1997) Targeted gene disruption reveals a leptin-independent role for the mouse beta3-adrenoceptor in the regulation of body composition. J Clin Invest 100(5):1098–1106

114. Green SA, Holt BD, Liggett SB (1992) Beta 1- and beta 2-adrenergic receptors display subtype-selective coupling to Gs. Mol Pharmacol 41(5):889–893

115. Levy FO, Zhu X, Kaumann AJ, Birnbaumer L (1993) Efficacy of beta 1-adrenergic receptors is lower than that of beta 2-adrenergic receptors. Proc Natl Acad Sci USA 90(22):10798–10802

β-Adrenergic Signal Transduction Defects in Heart Failure

Petra Schnabel, Markus Flesch, and Michael Böhm

The β-Adrenergic Signaling Pathway

In the mammalian heart, signaling through β-adrenergic receptors and the subsequent activation of the G protein–adenylyl cyclase signal transduction cascade is essential for the regulation of inotropy, chronotropy, dromotropy, lusitropy, and growth. The following chapter will give a review of the components generally involved in β-adrenergic signaling and of alterations in expression or function of these molecules in heart failure.

β-Adrenergic Receptors

β-Adrenergic receptors belong to the large family of G protein-coupled receptors. This family includes several hundred members characterized by a typical structure with an extracellular amino terminus, seven transmembrane domains, and an intracellular carboxy terminus (Gudermann et al. 1995). While the putative ligand-binding domain is formed by the amino terminus and certain portions of the transmembrane domains, the intracellular loops, particularly the third one, seem to be involved in the interaction with signal-transducing G proteins. The C-terminal portion of the receptors contain phosphorylation sites which serve as targets for protein kinase A (PKA), protein kinase C (PKC), and β-adrenergic receptor kinases (βARK). Three types of β-adrenergic receptors, designated β_1-, β_2-, and β_3-adrenoceptors, have been cloned from mammalian tissues until now (Dohlman et al. 1991; Gudermann et al. 1995). In the heart, the β_1-adrenoceptor-subtype is predominant, but functional coupling has also been demonstrated for the β_2-subtype. Several authors identified a third cardiac β-adrenergic receptor population. However, it is controversial whether these receptors are identical with the β_3-adrenoceptor present in adipose tissue as suggested by Gauthier et al. (1996). These authors suggest that β_3-adrenoceptors are expressed in the human heart and provide evidence that, in contrast to β_1- and β_2-adrenergic receptors, they mediate negative inotropic effects like G_i-coupled receptors. Other investigators (Evans et al. 1996; Kaumann and Molenaar 1996; Krief et al. 1993) also postulate the presence of a third β-adrenergic receptor population in the mammalian heart, but report it to be distinct from the β_3-adrenergic receptor cloned from adipose tissue. Cardiac β-adrenergic receptors are primarily activated by noradrenaline locally released from sympathetic nerve endings rather than circulating adrenaline. Noradrenaline exerts the highest affinity to the β_1-adrenoceptor subtype arguing in favor of the predominant physiological importance of this particular subtype.

β-Adrenergic receptor signaling can be desensitized at the level of the receptor, i.e., receptor expression or function can be reduced in response to prolonged or repeated receptor stimulation. Receptor expression is regulated over several hours, and a reduction of receptor mRNA and protein levels, i.e., receptor downregulation, can be due by a decrease in receptor synthesis or an increase in receptor degradation or sequestration into an intracellular compartment, a process which seems to be reversible (Pippig et al. 1995). In addition, β_2-adrenergic receptor number can be decreased by mRNA destabilization in response to agonist exposure (Hadcock et al. 1989). Destabilization of β_2-adrenergic receptor mRNA is associated with induction of proteins binding to adenine-uridine-rich regions in the 3' untranslated regions of receptor mRNAs (Port et al. 1992; Tholanikunnel et al. 1995). For the β_1-adrenergic receptor, a regulation of mRNA stability has not yet been shown. However, β_1-adrenoceptor downregulation has been suggested to be due to decreased transcriptional activity (Hosoda et al. 1994). Taken together, the data available have been obtained in different cellular systems and it is not possible to draw definitive conclusions concerning the mechanisms of β-adrenergic receptor downregulation in the mammalian heart. In contrast to receptor downregulation, i.e., changes in β-adrenoceptor expression, a loss of receptor function as a result of uncoupling from the signal-transducing G protein G_s can occur within a few seconds. This rapid process can be induced by receptor phosphorylation in the C-terminal domain by protein kinases A and C, and *β*-adrenergic receptor kinase (*β*ARK). Protein kinases A and C are activated by the second messenger molecules cAMP and diacyl glycerol, respectively. These second messengers are generated in response to activation of G protein-coupled receptors such as *β*- and *α*-adrenergic receptors, respectively. Receptor phosphorylation by PKA and PKC blocks the interaction of the receptor with the stimulatory G protein, G_s (Bouvier et al. 1987). A mechanism of highly specific homologous desensitization of *β*-adrenergic receptors is supplied by the *β*-adrenergic receptor kinase (*β*ARK), a serine/threonine kinase belonging to the family of G protein-coupled receptor kinases (GRKs; see Lefkowitz 1993 for review). There are two isoforms designated *β*ARK-1 and *β*ARK-2 (corresponding to GRK-2 and GRK-3 in the GRK terminology), both of which are expressed in the mammalian heart (Ungerer et al. 1994). *β*ARK phosphory-

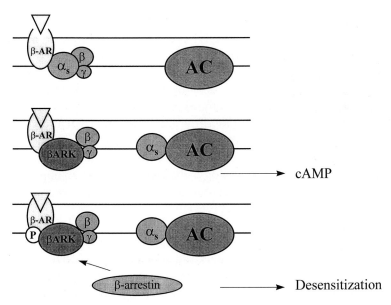

Fig. 1. Proposed mechanism of homologous receptor desensitization by *β*-adrenoceptor kinase (*β*ARK) and *β*-arrestin. For details, see text

lates agonist-liganded receptors, which thus become a substrate for β-arrestin, a cytosolic protein which binds to the receptor and leads to uncoupling from the stimulatory G protein, G_s. βARK itself is a cytosolic protein and requires translocation to the plasma membrane prior to enzymatic activity. There is evidence that membrane association is accomplished by interaction with G protein $\beta\gamma$-subunits (Pitcher et al. 1992), which takes place in the C-terminal region of the βARK polypeptide (Koch et al. 1993) and stimulates βARK activity (Inglese et al. 1992). There are two isoforms of β-arrestin referred to as β-arrestin-1 and β-arrestin-2, both of which are expressed in the mammalian heart. The predominant cardiac isoform is β-arrestin-1 (Ungerer et al. 1994) (Fig. 1).

Signal-Transducing G Proteins

Heterotrimeric G proteins couple the signals of many hormones, neurotransmitters, growth factors, and primary sensory stimuli from seven transmembrane-spanning receptors to intracellular effector moieties (see Birnbaumer et al. 1990 for review). Effectors can be enzymes such as adenylyl cyclase, phospholipase C, cGMP phosphodiesterase, or ion channels such as potassium and calcium channels. Heterotrimeric G proteins are composed of three distinct polypeptide chains designated α- (39–52 kDa), β- (35–36 kDa), and γ- (7–8 kDa) subunits. There is a considerable degree of diversity among the different subunits (Nürnberg et al. 1995; Simon et al. 1991). To date, the cDNAs of 16 α-, five β-, and ten γ-subunits have been cloned. The α-subunits are, according to their overall sequence homology, divided into four groups designated α_s, α_i, α_q, and α_{12}, each of them containing several members.

All known G proteins are activated and inactivated in a similar manner: an activated receptor interacts with the heterotrimeric G protein. This interaction triggers the replacement of GDP, which is bound to the α-subunit in the inactive state, by GTP. Subsequently, the heterotrimer dissociates into a free, GTP-liganded α-subunit and the $\beta\gamma$-dimer. Both α-subunits and $\beta\gamma$-dimers can interact with effectors such as phospholipase C and adenylyl cyclase. The activation cycle is terminated by the intrinsic GTPase activity of the *a*-subunit which cleaves the *a*-subunit-bound GTP into GDP and P_i. The GDP-bound *a*-subunit reassociates with the *βγ*-dimer to form the heterotrimer present in the inactive state (see Birnbaumer et al. 1990 for review).

Adenylyl cyclase is dually regulated by a_s and a_i proteins. a_s stimulates adenylyl cyclase and activates calcium channels. It is substrate to covalent modification by cholera toxin. The toxin cleaves NAD into nicotinamide and ADP-ribose and links the ADP-ribose moiety covalently to an arginine residue of the as polypeptide chain resulting in inhibition of the GTPase activity and thus constitutive activation of a_s. The human as gene has been mapped to chromosome 20 (Levine et al. 1991) and is composed of 13 exons and 12 introns. There are four splice variants generated by alternate use of exon 3 and two different 3′ splice sites of intron 3 which are functionally indistinguishable.

The family of adenylyl cyclase-inhibiting a_i proteins comprises three members, a_{i1}, a_{i2}, and a_{i3}. Each a_i-subunit is the product of

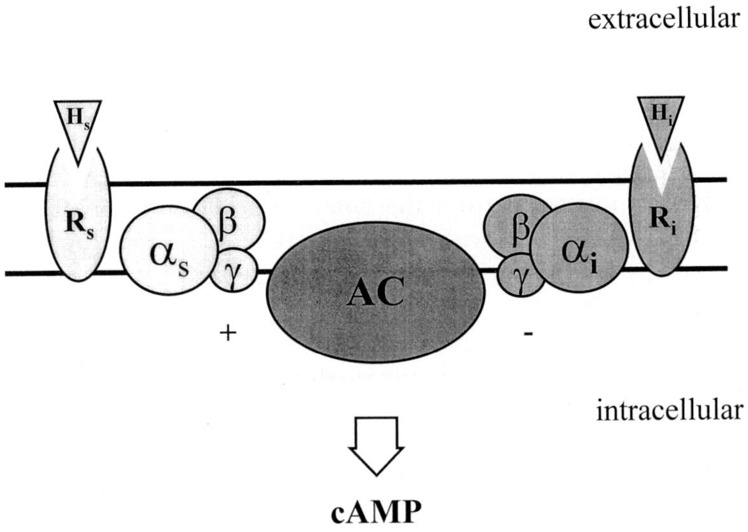

Fig. 2. Dual control of adenylyl cyclase (AC) via stimulatory (R_s) and inhibitory (R_i) cell surface receptors and stimulatory ($a_s βγ$) and inhibitory ($a_i bγ$) G proteins. *For details, see text*

a distinct gene (see Kaziro et al. 1991 for review). The rate of amino acid identity of these three genes is approximately 85%. The three human a_i genes are composed of eight coding exons and seven introns and have an identical exon–intron organization. In vitro, all three a_i-subunits inhibit adenylyl cyclase, but they are also able to interact with other effector systems such as potassium channels (see Birnbaumer 1990 for review). a_i Proteins are substrates to ADP-ribosylation by pertussis toxin, which covalently links ADP-ribose to a cysteine residue close to the C-terminus common to a_{i1}, a_{i2}, and a_{i3}. In contrast to a_s, which is constitutively activated, a_i proteins are uncoupled from the receptor by this modification. The a_i-subunit predominantly expressed in the mammalian heart is a_{i2}, although a_{i3} is also present (Böhm et al. 1990; Eschenhagen 1993). The significance of this molecular diversity within one tissue is not yet clear, and it is not known whether there is specificity concerning the interaction with certain cardiac receptors or adenylyl cyclase isozymes.

$\beta\gamma$-Subunits are important players in G protein-mediated signaling (see Clapham and Neer 1993 for review). The dimer remains tightly associated during the entire activation cycle of the G protein. β-Subunits are predicted to form coiled-coil structures in their amino-terminal region, which are stabilized a-helices important for protein–protein interactions, especially with the γ-subunit. The γ-subunits, which share a lower sequence homology than the β-subunits, are subject to a cascade of post-translational modifications (Wedegaertner et al. 1995). First, a cysteine residue four amino acids upstream from the C-terminus is isoprenylated. Second, the C-terminal three residues are cleaved by proteolysis. Third, carboxymethylation of the isoprenylated cysteine residue occurs. These steps are important for the function of the $\beta\gamma$-subunits. In rat heart, the expression of β_1, β_2, γ_3, γ_5, and γ_7 has been demonstrated (Hansen et al. 1995). However, it is not clear which combinations are formed in vivo and whether there is specificity of certain $\beta\gamma$-combinations for certain receptors, a-subunits, or effectors. Evidence of a high degree of specificity of $\beta\gamma$-interactions has been presented by Kleuss et al. (1991, 1992, 1993). An increasing number of effectors such as adenylyl cyclase, phospholipase C, βARK, phosphoinositide-3-kinase, and many others (see Nürnberg et al. 1995 for review) have been shown to be regulated by $\beta\gamma$-subunits in either a stimulatory or an inhibitory manner. In the mammalian heart, it has not yet been systematically investigated which $\beta\gamma$-dimers are formed. The regulation of adenylyl cyclase by G protein α- and $\beta\gamma$-subunits is reviewed in the following paragraph.

Adenylyl cyclase converts ATP into cyclic AMP, an intracellular second messenger molecule which is involved in the regulation of important cell functions such as metabolism and growth. Many of the actions of cAMP are mediated by cAMP-dependent protein kinases. In the heart, an increase of intracellular cAMP by adenylyl cyclase leads to activation of cAMP-dependent protein kinase A, which phosphorylates L-type calcium channels resulting in an increased trans-sarcolemmal calcium influx, increased sarcoplasmic reticulum calcium ATPase activity, and, consequently, increased contractility. Adenylyl cyclase activity is modulated in a stimulatory or inhibitory manner by extracellular signaling molecules such as hormones and neurotransmitters, which exert their action through seven transmembrane spanning receptors and G_s or G_i proteins, respectively.

Mammalian adenylyl cyclases are membrane-bound proteins with a short amino-terminal region (N), a hydrophobic domain (M1) predicted to cross the plasma membrane six times, a cytoplasmic domain (C1), a second hydrophobic domain with six transmembrane stretches (M2), and a C-terminal cytoplasmic domain (C2) (see Tang and Gilman 1992 for review). The cytoplasmic domains are highly conserved among the mammalian isozymes and between adenylyl and guanylyl cyclases and are required for catalytic activity.

Six distinct adenylyl cyclase isozymes designated AC-I to AC-VI have been cloned from mammalian tissues up until now (see Tang and Gilman 1992 for review). All of them are stimulated by α_s. In addition, AC-II and AC-IV are sensitive to stimulation by G protein $\beta\gamma$-subunits (Tang and Gilman 1991; Taussig et al. 1993): In contrast, AC-I is inhibited by $\beta\gamma$-subunits. AC-III, AC-V, and AC-VI isozymes are unaffected by $\beta\gamma$-subunits. The combinations of β- and γ-subunits forming dimers functional regarding adenylyl cyclase regulation are not yet identified. In contrast to phospholipase C activation, adenylyl cyclase activation by $\beta\gamma$-subunits is only observed in the presence of activated α_s. Thus, AC-II and AC-IV are molecular machines integrating coincident signals (Bourne and Nicoll 1993). Mammalian heart contains the adenylyl cyclase isozymes AC-IV (Gao and Gilman 1991), AC-V, and AC-VI (Tang and Gilman 1992). Thus, $\beta\gamma$-subunit-sensitive as well as -insensitive isozymes are present. The question whether myocardial adenylyl cyclase activity is stimulated or inhibited by free $\beta\gamma$-subunits has not yet been addressed directly. In general, α_s-, α_i-, and $\beta\gamma$-subunits are involved in the regulation of adenylyl cyclase. The exact molecular interactions taking place in mammalian myocardium remain to be identified.

Alterations of β-Adrenergic Signal Transduction in Heart Failure

Heart failure is characterized by inadequate cardiac output, which is unable to meet the demands of the body for oxygen and substrates. In order to maintain organ perfusion, the sympathetic nervous system is activated (Packer 1988). In heart failure, circulating norepinephrine levels are increased at rest (Cohn 1989) and during exercise (Francis et al. 1982). Moreover, norepinephrine is released locally from hearts in patients with heart failure (Swedberg et al. 1984).

β-Adrenergic Receptors

In the myocardium of patients with heart failure, myocardial β-adrenergic receptor density is markedly reduced (Bristow et al. 1982). This reduction is mainly due to reduction in the density of the β_1-adrenergic receptor subtype (Bristow et al. 1986; see Brodde 1996 for review), while the density of β_2-adrenergic receptors is unchanged. However, the stimulation of adenylyl cyclase via β_2-adrenergic receptors is impaired in patients with heart failure (Bristow et al. 1989). This functional uncoupling of β_2-adrenergic receptors might be due to the action of βARK, which induces uncoupling of β-adrenergic receptors from the downstream signaling molecules. Consistently, mRNA levels as well as enzyme activity of βARK are increased in the myocardium from patients with heart failure (Ungerer et al. 1993). There is a substantial increase of the βARK-1 and a moderate increase of the βARK-2 sub-

Table 1. Alterations of the *β*-adrenergic system in human heart failure

Alteration	Reference	Technique
Downregulation of β_1-AR	Bristow et al. (1982, 1986)	Radioligand binding
Uncoupling of β_2-AR	Bristow et al. (1989)	AC activity
Increase in *β*ARK	Ungerer et al. (1993, 1994)	RT-PCR
Increase in a_i (a_{i2})	Feldman et al. (1988)	Pertussis toxin labeling
	Neumann et al. (1988)	Pertussis toxin labeling
	Böhm et al. (1990)	Pertussis toxin labeling Western blotting
	Eschenhagen et al. (1992)	Northern blotting

type (Ungerer et al. 1994). In contrast, steady state levels of *β*-ar-restin-1 and *β*-arrestin-2 are similar in normal and failing human hearts (Ungerer et al. 1994). The activity of PKA is also not changed in human heart failure (Böhm et al. 1994). Taken to-gether, desensitization of the *β*-adrenergic system in human heart failure involves downregulation of β_1-adrenergic receptors and functional uncoupling of β_2-adrenergic receptors. The latter might be due to increased expression and activity of *β*ARK (Tab. 1).

The findings and hypotheses delineated above have been sup-ported by the generation of transgenic mice overexpressing com-ponents of the *β*-adrenergic system (see Rockman et al. 1996 for review).

Signal-Transducing G Proteins

G_s is the heterotrimeric G protein which couples *β*-adrenergic re-ceptors to adenylyl cyclase. a_s Can be visualized and quantified by cholera toxin-induced [^{32}P]ADP-ribosylation using [^{32}P]NAD as a substrate and subsequent separation on a SDS-polyacrylamide gel and autoradiography. Cholera toxin-induced [^{32}P]ADP-ribosylation of as is similar in human failing and nonfailing hearts (Feldman et al. 1988). However, the signals obtained by this technology are rather weak. Therefore, our group partially purified ARF (ADP-ri-bosylation factor), a cofactor of cholera toxin, from bovine brain cytosol and thus enhanced cholera toxin-induced [^{32}P]ADP-ribosylation of a_s in human left ventricular membranes (Schnabel et al. 1990). This method also revealed unchanged [^{32}P]ADP-ribosylation signals in heart failure. However, even this improved method of visualizing as is hampered by data suggesting that only a small portion of as present in myocardial membranes is ADP-ribosylated by cholera toxin (Insel and Ransnäs 1988). Levels of a_s mRNA have been reported to be similar (Eschenhagen et al. 1992) or increased (Feldman et al. 1989) in failing human hearts. Bioactivity of a_s was investigated by solubilization from myocardial membranes and reconstitution with S49 cyc$^-$ membranes. The cyc$^-$ mutant of S49 mouse lymphoma cells is genetically deficient of as. This method has also revealed unchanged a_s activity in heart failure as judged by unchanged isoprenaline- and Gpp(NH)p-stimulated adenylyl cyclase activity in the reconstituted lipid vesicles (Feldman et al. 1988). Taken together, the results obtained by different techniques and different authors strongly suggest unchanged amounts and bioactivity of a_s in human heart failure. However, in human heart failure due to Chagas cardiomyopathy (Morris et al. 1990) as well as in several animal models such as aortic banding in dogs (Longabaugh et al. 1988; Vatner et al. 1985) and hereditary cardiomyopathy in Syrian hamsters (Kessler et al. 1989), decreased as bioactivity was observed, indicating the dependence of the regulation of the β-adrenergic–G protein–adenylyl cyclase system on the species and the pathogenesis.

a_i Proteins can be visualized and quantified by pertussis toxin-induced [^{32}P]ADP-ribosyation. Several authors (Böhm et al. 1990; Feldman et al. 1988; Hershberger et al. 1991; Neumann et al. 1988) observed a substantial increase of pertussis toxin-induced [^{32}P]ADP-ribosylation of a_i in failing compared to nonfailing human hearts. However, a_i quantification by [^{32}P]ADP-ribosylation is hampered by possible endogenous ADP-ribosylation (Tanuma et al. 1988) or other kinds of covalent modification such as phosphorylation (Watanabe et al. 1988) at the C-terminus. In addition, several factors like $\beta\gamma$-subunits enhance ADP-ribosylation and thus differences in these factors might influence the results. Quantification of a_i by Western blotting using polyclonal rabbit antisera (Goldsmith et al. 1987) recognizing all a_i-subtypes has been done by several groups with discrepant results. Böhm et al. (1990)

found increased immunoreactivity in left ventricles from patients with dilated cardiomyopathy and unchanged amounts of αi in ischemic cardiomyopathy. Feldman et al. (1991) observed unchanged amounts of αi also in dilated cardiomyopathy. The reason for this discrepancy is not clear. The results of our group were confirmed by a radioimmunoassay with purified retinal transducin as standard and the $[^{125}I]$-labeled C-terminal decapeptide of transducin-α as tracer, revealing a marked increase of immunoreactive α_i proteins (Böhm et al. 1994). A differentiation between the different α_i-subtypes (α_{i2} and α_{i3} are expressed in the heart) is not possible with the antibodies applied. At the level of mRNA, a subtype-specific increase of α_{i2} has been demonstrated, while α_{i3} mRNA is similar in failing and nonfailing human hearts (Eschenhagen et al. 1993). At this point there is again a discrepancy with a very useful animal model, namely isoprenaline-treated rats. In the hearts of these animals, an increase of both α_{i2} and α_{i3} mRNA (Eschenhagen et al. 1992) is observed. The increase of α_{i2} mRNA was paralleled by an increased transcriptional rate of the α_{i2} gene as assessed by nuclear run-on assays performed with nuclear extracts from isoprenaline-treated rat cardiomyocytes (Müller et al. 1993). Thus, increased transcriptional activity contributes to the upregulation of α_{i2} in this system. The upregulation of α_i is not observed in S49 cyc⁻ or kin⁻ cells lacking or PKA, respectively, indicating that an intact G_s–adenylyl cyclase–PKA signaling cascade is required for this process in rat cardiomyocytes. In the human heart, there are no data available on this issue yet.

Although *β*-adrenergic receptors do not transduce their signals via G_i proteins, G_i influences the balance between stimulatory and inhibitory effects on adenylyl cyclase and might thus contribute to decreased adenylyl cyclase and inotropic response to *β*-adrenergic agonists. This hypothesis is supported by the finding that adenylyl cyclase activity of the failing human left ventricle (Feldman et al. 1988) is restored when the membranes are pretreated with pertussis toxin, which uncouples G_i from inhibitory receptors. In pertussis toxin-treated isolated human cardiomyocytes from patients with heart failure, isoprenaline-stimulated contractile force was restored to the level of cardiomyocytes from nonfailing hearts (Brown and Harding 1992). Taken together, it appears likely that the upregulation of α_{i2} contributes to the decreased inotropic response to β-adrenergic agonists and is of pathophysiological relevance in heart failure.

Adenylyl Cyclase

As mentioned above, adenylyl cyclase types IV, V, and VI are the isozymes present in the mammalian heart. Surprisingly, there are not many studies dealing with adenylyl cyclase isozyme expression patterns in the heart and qualitative or quantitative changes thereof in heart failure. In human heart failure due to dilated or ischemic cardiomyopathy, the mRNA of type V adenylyl cyclase, the predominant cardiac isozyme, is increased (Holmer et al. 1996). The mechanism of this increase has not yet been addressed. The observation suggests that adenylyl cyclase might not be impaired in heart failure, which is consistent with the previous observation (Böhm et al. 1990) that maximal adenylyl cyclase activity as assessed by stimulation with forskolin is not compromised in human heart failure. However, Holmer et al. (1996) only investigated adenylyl cyclase type V and not types IV and VI. In contrast, in pacing-induced heart failure in dogs, AV-V and AC-VI mRNA levels both are decreased (Ishikawa et al. 1994). Taken together, the data obtained in human myocardial tissue are not yet convincing enough to draw final conclusions on possible changes in adenylyl cyclase isoform expression.

Drug Action on the β-Adrenergic System

Downregulation of β-adrenergic receptors and increase of pertussis toxin substrates are observed not only in myocardial tissue homogenates, but also in isolated cardiomyocytes from neonatal rats treated with norepinephrine (Reithmann and Werdan 1989). In these cells, desensitization of the β-adrenergic signal transduction pathway can be prevented by the β-adrenergic antagonist propranolol, but not by the α-adrenergic antagonist prazosin. In the animal model of isoprenaline-treated rats (Eschenhagen et al. 1992), the β-adrenergic antagonists can also prevent desensitization. In spontaneously hypertensive rats, which also exhibit desen-

sitization of the *β*-adrenergic system, angiotensin-converting enzyme inhibitors (Böhm et al. 1995) can also resensitize the *β*-adre-
nergic system (Böhm et al. 1995 a,b,c), indicating cross-talk between these two neuroendocrine systems. In human heart failure,
metoprolol treatment has also been shown to increase *β*-adrener-
gic receptor density in endomyocardial biopsies and to improve
hemodynamic responses to catecholamines in patients with dilated cardiomyopathy (Heilbrunn et al. 1989). The increase of α_i
has also been shown to be reversed by metoprolol treatment in
patients with dilated cardiomyopathy (Sigmund et al. 1996). Inter-
estingly, an increase in *β*-adrenergic receptor density is only observed in patients treated with metoprolol and not in patients
treated with the vasodilating *β*-blocker carvedilol, although hemodynamics improve similarly in the two groups (Gilbert et al.
1993). The molecular mechanisms of these differential responses
are not yet clarified.

Perspectives

The diversity of signal transduction molecules involved in *β*-adre-
nergic signal transduction is considerable, and so are the possibi-
lities of interactions and cross-talk between them. Even today, it is
not clear which signaling molecules are expressed in cardiac tissue and particularly in the cardiomyocyte. Moreover, the observation of alterations of signal transduction components are purely
descriptive and do not automatically establish a pathophysiological role. To this end, in vitro and in vivo gene transfer techniques
and transgenic methodologies will have to be applied to a larger
extent. However, the research done on the *β*-adrenergic system so
far has already had an impact on the treatment of patients with
heart failure: Based on the observation that *β*-adrenoceptors are
downregulated in the presence of high catecholamine levels and
can be upregulated in the presence of *β*-adrenoceptor antagonists,
β-blockers, formerly considered contraindicated in heart failure,
are now a well established therapeutic agent improving exercise
tolerance and prognosis of patients with heart failure (see Cleland
et al. 1996 for review).

References

Birnbaumer L, Abramowitz J, Brown AM (1990) Receptor–effector coupling by G proteins. Biochim Biophys Acta 1031:163–224

Böhm M, Gierschik P, Jakobs KH, Pieske B, Schnabel P, Ungerer M, Erdmann E (1990) Increase of Giα in human hearts with dilated but not ischemic cardiomyopathy. Circulation 82:1249–1265

Böhm M, Reiger B, Schwinger RHG, Erdmann E (1994) cAMP-concentrations, cAMP-dependent protein kinase activity and phospholamban in nonfailing and failing myocardium. Cardiovasc Res 28:1713–1719

Böhm M, Gräbel C, Knorr A, Erdmann E (1995a) Treatment in hypertensive cardiac hypertrophy, I. Neuropeptide Y and β-adrenoceptors. Hypertension 25:954–961

Böhm M, Gräbel C, Flesch M, Knorr A, Erdmann E (1995b) Treatment in hypertensive cardiac hypertrophy, II. Postreceptor events. Hypertension 25:962–970

Böhm M, Castellano M, Agabiti-Rosei E, Flesch M, Paul M, Erdmann E (1995c) Dose-dependent dissociation of ACE-inhibitor effects on blood pressure, cardiac hypertrophy, and beta-adrenergic signal transduction. Circulation 92:3006–3013

Bourne HR, Nicoll RA (1993) Molecular machines integrate coincident synaptic signals. Cell/Neuron 72/12:65–75

Bouvier M, Leeb-Lundberg LMF, Benovic JL, Caron MG, Lefkowitz RJ (1987) Regulation of adrenergic receptor function by phosphorylation. II. Effects of agonist occupancy on phosphorylation of α_1- and β_2-adrenergic receptors by protein kinase C and the cyclic AMP-dependent protein kinase. J Biol Chem 262:3106–3113

Bristow MR, Ginsburg R, Minobe W, Cubicciotti RS, Sageman WS, Lurie K, Billingham ME, Harrison DC, Stinson EB (1982) Decreased catecholamine sensitivity and β-adrenergic receptor density in failing human hearts. N Engl J Med 307:205–211

Brodde OE (1996) β-Adrenergic receptors in failing human myocardium. Basic Res Cardiol 91(Suppl. 2):35–40

Brown LA, Harding SE (1992) The effect of pertussis toxin on β-adrenoceptor responses in isolated cardiac myocytes from noradrenaline-treated guinea pigs and patients with heart failure. Br J Pharmacol 106:115–122

Clapham DE, Neer EJ (1993) New roles for G-protein βγ-dimers in transmembrane signaling. Nature 365:403–406

Cleland JGF, Bristow MR, Erdmann E, Remme WJ, Swedberg K, Waagstein F (1996) Beta-blocking agent in heart failure. Eur Heart J 17:1629–1639

Cohn JN (1989) The sympathetic nervous system in heart failure. J Cardiovasc Pharmacol 14(Suppl. 5):57–61

Dohlman HG, Thorner J, Caron MG, Lefkowitz RJ (1991) Model systems for the study of seven-transmembrane-segment receptors. Annu Rev Biochem 60:653–688

Eschenhagen T (1993) G proteins in the heart. Cell Biol Int 17:723–749

Eschenhagen T, Mende U, Nose M, Schmitz W, Scholz H, Haverich A, Hirt S, Döring V, Kalmar P, Höppner W, Seitz HJ (1992) Increased messenger RNA level of the inhibitory G-protein *α*-subunit Giα2 in human end-stage heart failure. Circ Res 70:688–696

Eschenhagen T, Mende U, Nose M, Schmitz W, Scholz H, Schulte am Esch J, Warnholz A (1992) Long term *β*-adrenoceptor-mediated upregulation of Giα- and Goα-mRNA levels and pertussis toxin sensitive G-proteins in rat heart. Mol Pharmacol 42:773–783

Evans BA, Papaioannou M, Bonazzi VR, Summers RJ (1996) Expression of *β*-adrenoceptor mRNA in rat tissues. Br J Pharmacol 117:210–216

Feldman AM, Cates AE, Veazey WB, Hershberger RE, Bristow MR, Baughman KL, Baumgartner WA, Van Dop C (1988) Increase in the 40,000-mol wt pertussis toxin substrate (G-protein) in the failing human heart. J Clin Invest 82: 189-197

Feldman AM, Cates AE, Bristow MR, Van Dop C (1989) Altered expression of the *α*-subunits of G-proteins in failing human hearts. J Mol Cell Cardiol 21:359–365

Feldman AM, Jackson DG, Bristow MR, Cates AE, Van Dop C (1991) Immunodetectable levels of the inhibitory guanine nucleotide-binding regulatory proteins in failing human heart. J Mol Cell Cardiol 23:439–452

Francis GS, Goldsmith SR, Ziesche SM, Cohn JN (1982) Response of plasma norepinephrine and epinephrine to dynamic exercise in patients with congestive heart failure. Am J Cardiol 49:1152–1159

Gao B, Gilman AG (1991) Cloning and expression of a widely distributed (type IV) adenylyl cyclase. Proc Natl Acad Sci USA 88:10178–10182

Gauthier C, Tavernier G, Charpentier F, Langin D, Le Marec H (1996) Functional *β*3-adrenoceptor in the human heart. J Clin Invest 98:556–562

Gilbert EM, Olsen SL, Renlund DG, Bristow MR (1993) Beta-adrenergic receptor regulation and left ventricular function in idiopathic dilated cardiomyopathy. Am J Cardiol 71:23C-29C

Goldsmith P, Gierschik P, Milligan G, Unson CG, Vinitsky R, Malech HL, Spiegel AM (1987) Antibodies directed against synthetic peptides distinguish between GTP-binding proteins in neutrophils and brain. J Biol Chem 262:14683–14688

Gudermann T, Nürnberg B, Schultz G (1995) Receptors and G proteins as primary components of transmembrane signal transduction. Part 1. G-protein-coupled receptors: structure and function. J Mol Med 73:51–63

Hadcock JR, Wang H, Malbon CC (1989) Agonist-induced destabilization of *β*-adrenergic receptor mRNA attenuation of glucocorticoid-induced up-regulation of *β*-adrenergic receptors. J Biol Chem 264:19928–19933

Hansen CA, Schroering AG, Robishaw JD (1995) Subunit expression of signal transducing G proteins in cardiac tissue: implications for phospholipase C-*β* regulation. J Mol Cell Cardiol 27:471–484

Heilbrunn SM, Shah P, Bristow MR, Valantine HA, Ginsburg R, Fowler MB (1989) Increased *β*-receptor density and improved hemodynamic response to catecholamine stimulation during long-term metoprolol therapy in heart failure from dilated cardiomyopathy. Circulation 79:483–490

Hershberger RE, Feldman AM, Bristow MR (1991) A1-adenosine receptor inhibition of adenylate cyclase in failing and nonfailing human myocardium. Circulation 83:1343–1351

Holmer SR, Eschenhagen T, Nose M, Riegger GAJ (1996) Expression of adenylyl cyclase and G-protein beta subunit in end-stage human heart failure. J Cardiac Failure 2:279–283

Hosoda K, Feussner GK, Rydelek-Fitzgerald L, Fishman PH, Duman RS (1994) Agonist and cyclic AMP-mediated regulation of β_1-adrenergic receptor mRNA and gene transcription in rat C6 glioma cells. J Neurochem 63:1635–1645

Inglese J, Koch WJ, Caron MG, Lefkowitz RJ (1992) Isoprenylation in regulation of signal transduction by G-protein-coupled receptor kinases. Nature 359:147–150

Insel PA, Ransnäs LA (1988) G-proteins and cardiovascular disease. Circulation 78:1511–1513

Ishikawa Y, Sorota S, Kiuchi K, Shannon RP, Komamura K, Katsushika S, Vatner DE, Vatner SF, Homcy CJ (1994) Downregulation of adenylyl cyclase types V and VI mRNA levels in pacing-induced heart failure in dogs. J Clin Invest 93:2224–2229

Kaumann AJ, Molenaar P (1996) Differences between the third cardiac β-adrenoceptor and the colonic β_3-adrenoceptor in the rat. Br J Pharmacol 118:2085–2098

Kaziro Y, Itoh H, Kozasa T, Nakafuku M, Satoh T (1991) Structure and function of signal-transducing GTP-binding proteins. Annu Rev Biochem 60:349–400

Kessler PD, Cates AE, Van Dop C, Feldman AM (1989) Decreased bioactivity of the guanine nucleotide-binding protein that stimulates adenylate cyclase in hearts from cardiomyopathic Syrian hamsters. J Clin Invest 84:244–252

Kleuss C, Hescheler J, Ewel C, Rosenthal W, Schultz G, Wittig B (1991) Assignment of G-protein subtypes to specific receptors inducing inhibition of calcium currents. Nature 353:43–48

Kleuss C, Scherübl H, Hescheler J, Schultz G, Wittig B (1992) Different β-subunits determine G-protein interaction with transmembrane receptors. Nature 358:424–426

Kleuss C, Scherübl H, Hescheler J, Schultz G, Wittig B (1993) Selectivity in signal transduction determined by γ subunits of heterotrimeric G proteins. Science 259:832–834

Koch WJ, Inglese J, Stone WC, Lefkowitz RJ (1993) The binding site for the $\beta\gamma$ subunits of heterotrimeric G proteins on the β-adrenergic receptor kinase. J Biol Chem 268:8256–8260

Krief S, Lönnqvist F, Raimbault S, Baude B, Van Spronsen A, Arner P, Strosberg AD, Ricquier D, Emorine LJ (1993) Tissue distribution of β_3-adrenergic receptor mRNA in man. J Clin Invest 91:344–349

Lefkowitz RJ (1993) G protein-coupled receptor kinases. Cell 74:409–412

Levine MA, Modi WS, O'Brien SJ (1991) Mapping of the gene encoding the α subunit of the stimulatory G protein of adenylyl cyclase (GNAS1) to 20q13.2–q13.3 in human by in situ hybridization. Genomics 11:478–479

Longabaugh JP, Vatner DE, Vatner SF, Homcy CJ (1988) Decreased stimulatory guanosine triphosphate binding protein in dogs with pressure overload left ventricular failure. J Clin Invest 81:420–424

Morris SA, Tanowitz H, Wittner M, Bilezilian JP (1990) Pathophysiological insights into the cardiomyopathy of Chagas' disease. Circulation 82:1900–1909

Neumann J, Scholz H, Döring V, Schmitz W, v. Meyerinck L, Kalmar P (1988) Increase in myocardial Gi-proteins in heart failure. Lancet II:936–937

Nürnberg B, Gudermann T, Schultz G (1995) Receptors and G proteins as primary components of transmembrane signal transduction. Part 2. G proteins: structure and function. J Mol Med 73:123–132

Packer M (1988) Neurohormonal interactions and adaptations in congestive heart failure. Circulation 77:721–730

Pippig S, Andexinger S, Lohse MJ (1995) Sequestration and recycling of β₂-adrenergic receptors permit receptor resensitization. Mol Pharmacol 47:666–676

Pitcher JA, Inglese J, Higgins JB, Kim C, Benovic JL, Kwatra MM, Caron MG, Lefkowitz RJ (1992) Role of βγ subunits of G proteins in targeting the β-adrenergic receptor kinase to membrane-bound receptors. Science 257:1264–1267

Port JD, Huang LJ, Malbon CC (1992) β-Adrenergic agonists that down-regulate receptor mRNA up-regulate a Mr 35,000 protein(s) that selectively binds to β-adrenergic receptor mRNAs. J Biol Chem 267:24103–24108

Reithmann C, Werdan K (1989) Noradrenaline-induced desensitization in cultured heart cells as a model for the defects of adenylate cyclase system in severe heart failure. Naunyn Schmiedeberg's Arch Pharmacol 339:138–144

Rockman HA, Koch WJ, Milano CA, Lefkowitz RJ (1996) Myocardial β-adrenergic receptor signaling in vivo: insights from transgenic mice. J Mol Med 74:489–495

Schnabel P, Böhm M, Gierschik P, Jakobs KH, Erdmann E (1990) Improvement of cholera toxin-catalyzed ADP-ribosylation by endogenous ADP-ribosylation factor from bovine brain provides evidence for unchanged amounts of Gsα in failing human myocardium. J Mol Cell Cardiol 22:73–82

Sigmund M, Jakob H, Becker H, Hanrath P, Schumacher C, Eschenhagen T, Schmitz W, Scholz H, Steinfath M (1996) Effects of metoprolol on myocardial β-adrenoceptors and Giα-proteins in patients with congestive heart failure. Eur J Clin Pharmacol 51:127–132

Simon MI, Strathmann MP, Gautam N (1991) Diversity of G proteins in signal transduction. Science 252:802–808

Swedberg K, Viquerat C, Rouleau JL, Roizen M, Atherton B, Parmley WW, Chatterjee K (1984) Comparison of myocardial catecholamine balance in chronic congestive heart failure and in angina pectoris without failure. Am J Cardiol 54:783–786

Tang WJ, Gilman AG (1991) Type-specific regulation of adenylyl cyclase by G protein $\beta\gamma$ subunits. Science 254:1500–1503

Tang WJ, Gilman AG (1992) Adenylyl cyclases. Cell 70:869–872

Tanuma S, Kawashima K, Endo H (1988) Eukaryotic mono (ADP) ribosyltransferase that ADP-ribosylates GTP-binding regulatory Gi*α* protein. J Biol Chem 263:5485–5489

Taussig R, Quarmby LM, Gilman AG (1993) Regulation of purified type I and type II adenylyl cyclases by G protein $\beta\gamma$ subunits. J Biol Chem 268:9–12

Tholanikunnel BG, Granneman JG, Malbon CC (1995) The Mr 35,000 *β*-adrenergic receptor mRNA-binding protein binds transcripts of G-protein-linked receptors which undergo agonist-induced destabilization. J Biol Chem 270:12787–12793

Ungerer M, Böhm M, Elce JS, Erdmann E, Lohse MJ (1993) Altered expression of *β*-adrenergic receptor kinase and β_1-adrenergic receptors in the failing human heart. Circulation 87:454–463

Ungerer M, Parruti G, Böhm M, Puzicha M, DeBlasi A, Erdmann E, Lohse MJ (1994) Expression of *β*-arrestins and *β*-adrenergic receptor kinases in the failing human heart. Circ Res 74:206–213

Vatner DE, Vatner SF, Fujii AM, Homcy CJ (1985) Loss of high affinity cardiac beta-adrenergic receptors in dogs with heart failure. J Clin Invest 76:2259–2264

Watanabe Y, Imaizumi T, Misaki N, Iwankura K, Yoshiba H (1988) Effects of phosphorylation of inhibitory GTP-binding protein by cyclic AMP-dependent protein kinase on its ADP-ribosylation by pertussis toxin, islet activating protein. FEBS Lett 236:372–374

Wedegaertner PB, Wilson PT, Bourne HR (1995) Lipid modifications of trimeric G proteins. J Biol Chem 270:503–506

β-Blocker Treatment of Chronic Heart Failure

C. Maack and M. Böhm

Introduction

Congestive heart failure is a major public health problem in most Western countries. In the United States, approximately 3 million people suffer from heart failure, 10% of whom are admitted to hospital each year [1]. Although in recent decades considerable advances in medical therapy have been achieved, especially by angiotensin-converting enzyme (ACE) inhibitors [2, 3], the mortality rate of heart failure still remains very high. In patients of New York Heart Association (NYHA) functional class II, there is a mortality rate of about 10% per year [4]. In order to improve this poor prognosis, additional pharmacological interventions to counteract the pathophysiological changes occurring in heart failure are still important.

Waagstein et al. (1975) were the first to treat patients with idiopathic dilated cardiomyopathy (IDC) with β-blockers in a small open trial [5]. They observed improvements in exercise tolerance and ventricular function and a reduction of heart size in these patients. Due to their negative inotropic actions, β-blockers were formerly not considered to be an appropriate treatment of heart failure. However, in 1979, in a retrospective analysis using matched historical controls, Swedberg et al. [6] suggested that β-blockers have a favorable effect on mortality in patients with heart failure. In 1980, these authors reported deleterious effects of β-blocker withdrawal and subsequent improvement after readministration in a group of 15 patients with IDC [7]. In another noncontrolled study of patients with IDC, this group reported that long-term (6–62 months) β-blockade resulted in an improvement in systolic and diastolic myocardial function and functional class [8]. These favorable initial studies have spawned a number of randomized double-blinded, placebo-controlled trials of heart failure investigating the effects of β-blockers on various hemodynamic factors, symptoms, functional class, exercise capacity and survival.

Pathophysiology of the β-Adrenergic System and Mechanisms of β-Receptor Blockade

In the early stages of heart failure several neuroendocrine mechanisms beneficial in acute hemodynamic shock are activated via maintenance of arterial blood pressure and blood flow to vital organs, thereby supplying these organs with sufficient amounts of oxygen. When chronically activated, these compensatory mechanisms, i.e., activation of the renin-angiotensin-aldosterone-system and the sympathetic nervous system, have a negative impact on cardiac function.

Plasma norepinephrine levels are chronically elevated in patients with heart failure, and the extent of elevation correlates with their poor prognosis [9]. The resulting increased stimulation of the β-adrenergic system leads to a desensitization of the adenylyl cyclase of the heart [10], which is caused by a decrease in β-adrenoceptor density on the surface of the cardiac myocytes [11], increased expression of the α-subunit of the inhibitory G-protein ($G_{i\alpha}$) [12] and phosphorylation of the receptors by increased activity and expression of the β–adrenoceptor kinase (βARK) [13]. The functional relevance of these cellular changes is reflected by a decreased response of the heart to catecholamines in vitro [12] and in vivo [14]. Furthermore, chronic β-adrenergic activation causes an increase in heart rate, which leads to reduced myocardial blood flow due to a shortened coronary vascular diastolic perfusion time. This has a negative impact on the balance of myocardial energy expenditure. The catecholamine-induced increase in calcium influx contributes to the high energy expenditure and leads to intracellular acidosis with impairment of oxydation phosphorylation [15] as well as activation of calcium-dependent proteases, which might contribute to the development of myocardial necrosis. The detrimental effect of persistent tachycardia on myocardial function is documented by the fact that in several animal models, heart failure can be induced by rapid left ventricular pacing. In normal human hearts, a rise in stimulation frequency is followed by an increase in cardiac contractility. This positive force-frequency relationship is blunted in the failing human heart, which can be observed in in-vivo [16] and in-vitro [17] experiments. Thus, tachycardia results in decreased myocardial contractility of the failing human heart.

These mechanisms clearly indicate the detrimental effects of chronic sympathetic activation on cardiac function and are a rationale for *β*-blocker therapy in patients with heart failure, as these compounds intervene with the pathophysiological changes that occur in heart failure. An overview of the most common agents used in patients with heart failure and their pharmacological properties is given in Table 1. Metoprolol and bisoprolol have a higher affinity to the $β_1$- than to the $β_2$-adrenoceptor. As in human heart, the majority of the *β*-receptors consists of the $β_1$-receptor population, with these agents exerting their pharmacological actions primarily in the heart. Adverse effects, such as bronchoconstriction or worsening of peripheral arterial disease, are mainly due to the blockade of $β_2$-receptors and thus occur to a smaller degree with these selective compounds. Carvedilol and bucindolol are nonselective *β*-blockers, but in addition to *β*-blockade these agents cause peripheral vasodilatation. In the case of carvedilol this is due to vascular *α*-adrenoceptor blockade, whereas in the case of bucindolol such action is adrenoceptor-independent. None of the listed agents exert intrinsic sympathomimetic activity (ISA). Partial agonists that exert ISA, like xamoterol, can increase heart rate and contractility to a small degree through weak stimulation of adenylyl cyclase.

Table 1. *Anti*oxidant properties in heart failure

	$β_1$-Selectivity	Vasodilatation	*α*-Receptor-antagonism	Antioxidant properties
Bisoprolol	++	–	–	–
Bucindolol	–	+	–	–
Carvedilol	(+)	+	+	+
Metoprolol	++	–	–	–

The application of β-blockers leads to a reduced heart rate, resulting in lower myocardial energy expenditure [18], prolonged diastolic filling [19] and increased effective myocardial blood flow due to prolonged coronary vascular diastolic perfusion time [20]. The importance of reducing heart rate is documented by the fact that therapy with xamoterol led to an increase in mortality in patients with severe heart failure. In these patients, especially at night, a higher heart rate was observed due to the intrinsic sympathomimetic activity of this agent [21].

Furthermore, plasma norepinephrine levels are reduced by β-blockers [22], but only carvedilol was shown to reduce cardiac norepinephrine release [23]. However, in both cases the myocardium is protected from the cardiotoxic effects of norepinephrine [24, 25]. In contrast to carvedilol therapy, metoprolol therapy caused an increase in left ventricular β-adrenoceptor density [26] and downregulated the increased expression of the G-protein [27]. This indicates that the two agents differ in β-adrenoceptor interaction [28]. However, it is unlikely that β-adrenoceptor density plays a crucial role in proper ventricular function, as left ventricular ejection fraction can be improved by carvedilol therapy (Fig. 1). In addition, a decreased β-receptor density can be upregulated within hours to days [29], whereas functional improvement usually does not occur until 3 months after the onset of β-blocker therapy [30].

Thus, one should consider other mechanisms contributing to the improvement of ventricular function. Kukin et al. [31] compared the effects of metoprolol and the combination of metoprolol and doxazosin (α-blocker) on ventricular function and hemodynamics in patients with heart failure in order to assess the relevance of α-receptor blockade. After 6 weeks of therapy a marked decline in vascular resistance and an increase in cardiac index were observed (Fig. 2). These beneficial effects on hemodynamics did not differ among the two groups. Thus, α-receptor blockade (i.e., by carvedilol) appears to have no crucial impact on hemodynamics in long-term therapy.

Of the listed compounds (Table 1), only carvedilol exerts antioxidant activity. The ability of carvedilol to prevent oxygen free radical damage or to scavenge free radicals directly was demonstrated by several in-vitro experiments [32, 33]. Oxygen free radicals occur not only in the reperfusion of ischemic myocardium ("myocardial stunning") [34], but also, in the plasma of patients with heart failure, an increased amount of malondialdehydes as an indicator of lipid peroxidation due to free radicals was observed, whereas the plasma thiol concentration, an indicator of the oxidative status of the extracellular environment, was significantly reduced compared to normal controls (Fig. 3) [35]. Both parameters correlated with an impaired cardiac function [35]. Oxygen free radicals have been implicated in the pathogenesis of vascular smooth muscle cell proliferation. Both in-vitro [36] and in-vivo [37] experiments demonstrated a concentration-dependent inhibi-

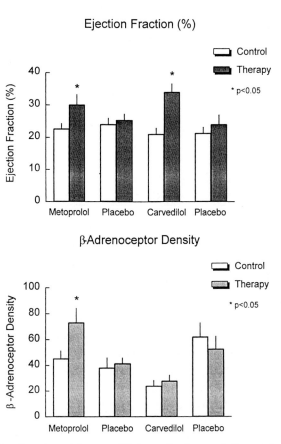

Fig. 1. Effects of metoprolol, carvedilol or placebo on left ventricular ejection fraction and *β*-adrenoceptor density in patients with heart failure [from 26]

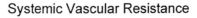

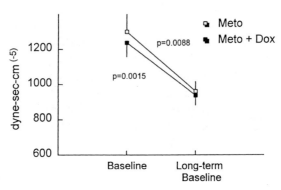

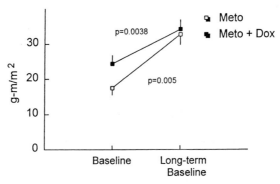

Fig. 2. Effects of β- or β- plus α-blockade in patients with heart failure [from 31]

tion of vascular smooth muscle cell proliferation by carvedilol. Thus, carvedilol treatment delayed the progression of coronary atheromas and altered vascular remodeling processes that occur in chronic heart failure caused by ischemic heart disease. Taken together, the multiple experimental data suggest an explanation for the beneficial effects of β-blockers observed in clinical trials, which ultimately comprise the crucial criterion for successful treatment of heart failure.

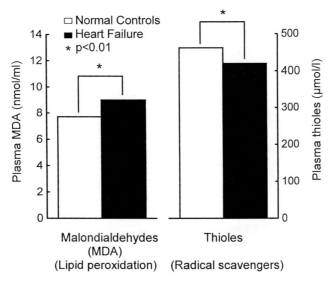

Fig. 3. Amount of oxygen free radical damage (lipid peroxidation) and free radical scavengers in the plasma of patients with heart failure [from 35]

Aims of Heart Failure Treatment and Its Evaluation

The objectives of the treatment of heart failure can be defined as prolonging active life and improving quality of life [38]. To achieve these goals, major adverse events should be prevented, such as hospitalization or recurrent myocardial infarction. Preventing the progression of cardiac dysfunction is an integral part of achieving these aims. In order to estimate the success of heart failure treatment, several subjective and objective parameters can be used. Among the subjective parameters are a clinical assessment of functional class (NYHA scores) and general assessment by the physician or patient. The objective parameters consist of the assessment of certain hemodynamic parameters, such as arterial blood pressure, heart rate, ventricular ejection fraction and volumina, but also of the determination of major adverse events, such as hospitalization, recurrent myocardial infarction, need for cardiac transplantation and death. Finally, the efficacy and tolerability of a drug can be assessed by the "dropout rate" in large clinical trials, which is an indicator of the patients' compliance.

Subjective Parameters

Most clinical trials with β_1-selective blockers demonstrated an improvement of symptoms. Metoprolol treatment significantly improved NYHA functional class in patients with idiopathic dilated cardiomyopathy (MDC study) [39] as well as ischemic cardiomyopathy (ICM) [40]. This also holds true for bisoprolol in a trial of 641 patients with both IDC and ICM (CIBIS I) [41]. As a nonselective β-blocker with vasodilatatory properties, bucindolol failed to improve NYHA functional class. It must be taken into account, however, that these studies [42, 43] were only of 3 months duration. This period of time can be considered too short to improve symptoms of heart failure by a β-blocking agent (see also below). The largest trials with more than 1000 patients altogether have been carried out with carvedilol. The most important of these are the US Carvedilol Heart Failure Study Group (US trials) [44] and the Australia-New Zealand Heart Failure Research Collaboratory Group (ANZ) [45]. In the US trials and in most of the smaller trials, a significant improvement in NYHA functional class was noted. In contrast, the ANZ revealed no significant improvement in NYHA functional class after 18 months of treatment with carvedilol.

Another indicator for symptoms of heart failure in the large clinical trials is the "dropout rate". This rate describes the number of patients who terminate participation in a controlled trial due to worsening of heart failure or adverse responses to a compound. In the US trials this dropout rate was significantly lower in the carvedilol group (5.5%) compared to placebo (8%). The MDC study revealed a comparable result for metoprolol (14% vs 21.4%).

Objective Parameters

Hemodynamics

By inhibiting the effects of catecholamines on cardiac *β*-adrener-
gic receptors, *β*-blockers are potential negative inotropic compounds, and thus contraindication has been suggested in patients
with heart failure. Waagstein et al. [46] compared acute and long-
term (6 months) effects of metoprolol treatment in patients with
heart failure. Figure 4 gives an overview of the results. After acute
administration of 5 mg of metoprolol intravenously, a significant
decrease in heart rate and a slight reduction of systolic blood

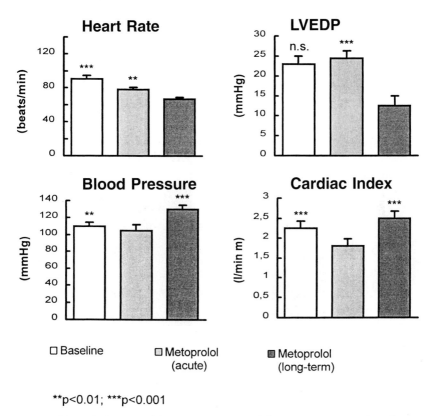

**p<0.01; ***p<0.001

Fig. 4. Effect of short- and long-term metoprolol treatment on various hemodynamic parameters [from 46]

pressure were observed, resulting in a significant decrease in cardiac index. Left ventricular enddiastolic pressure (LVEDP), an indicator for cardiac preload, rose consecutively. These changes in
hemodynamics are typical effects of a negative inotropic compound. In contrast, after 6 months of long-term therapy with initial doses of 5 mg of metoprolol and a slow uptitration to doses of
2×50 or even 2×100 mg, the hemodynamic situation changed completely. Despite a further decrease in heart rate, systolic blood
pressure and cardiac index increased significantly, resulting in a
pronounced decrease in LVEDP. These results indicate two things:
first, in long-term treatment the negative inotropic effect of the β-
blocker converts into maintenance of contractility; second, the results clearly demonstrate that high initial doses or uncautious uptitration of doses might lead to forward failure with decreased cardiac output or to backward failure with pulmonary edema and
elevated left ventricular filling pressures. Thus, β-blocker therapy
in patients with heart failure must be initiated very carefully and
should be controlled by a specialist.

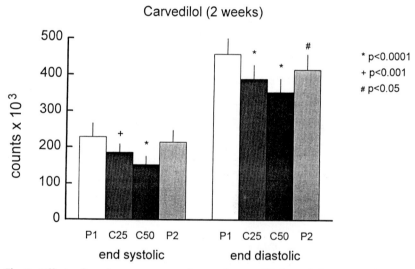

Fig. 5. Effect of various concentrations of carvedilol on left ventricular volumes in patients with stable angina pectoris. Patients entered a 2-week phase
taking placebo (P1). They then received carvedilol, 25 (C25) and then 50 mg
(C50) twice daily for two weeks on each dose, followed by another 2-week
placebo phase (P2) [from 47]

As early as 1987 comparable results were obtained in patients with stable angina pectoris who were treated with carvedilol. Lahiri et al. [47] observed a concentration-dependent decrease in endsystolic as well as enddiastolic volumes (Fig. 5). Withdrawal of carvedilol resulted in a subsequent increase in these parameters. As these data were achieved as early as 2 weeks after the onset of therapy, the *a*-receptor-blocking properties with subsequent vasodilatation may be responsible for this relatively acute reduction of pre- and afterload. These pharmacological properties of carvedilol might be of particular importance during the initiation and titration period of treatment, as this agent might be better tolerated due to its acute hemodynamic effects.

Ventricular Function and Remodeling

Although there is evidence for the development of tolerance to the vasodilating effects of *a*-receptor-blocking agents [48, 49], 12 months of carvedilol treatment in patients with heart failure demonstrated a progredient-positive impact on left ventricular volumes [50]. In a substudy of the ANZ trial of carvedilol in patients with heart failure due to ischemic heart disease, the effects of this treatment on left ventricular (LV) endsystolic and enddiastolic volumes and on LV ejection fraction were determined. Despite a basal treatment including ACE inhibitors, there was a continuous increase in LV endsystolic and enddiastolic volume index. In contrast, in patients receiving carvedilol, these parameters decreased significantly compared to controls (Fig. 6). Left ventricular ejection fraction increased by 4.9% in the carvedilol group compared with the placebo group, in which this parameter remained unaffected. These data suggest that in patients with heart failure, progressive left ventricular dilatation can occur despite a lack of deterioration of LV ejection fraction. These observations are in accordance with earlier results from patients after myocardial infarction [51]. In these patients left ventricular volumes were identified as important prognostic markers with regard to mortality [52, 53]. In studies on patients after myocardial infarction the ACE-inhibitor captopril was shown to attenuate left ventricular dilatation [54] and reduce mortality [55]. The causal relationship between

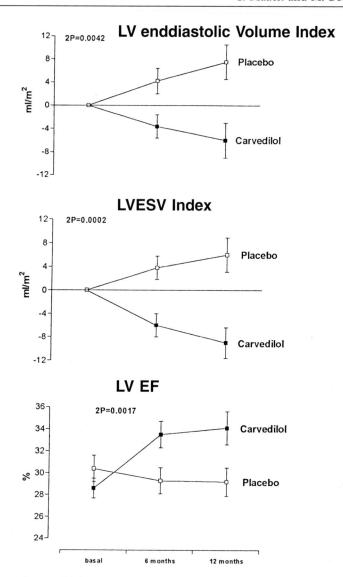

Fig. 6. Effect of carvedilol treatment on left ventricular volume indexes and ejection fraction in patients with chronic heart failure [from 45]

ventricular dilatation and mortality could be due to the observation that ventricular remodeling may result in both pump failure and sudden death [56]. These results clearly suggest the important role of ventricular remodeling in the development of heart failure after ischemic events. Hence, when considering the effect of intervention on left ventricular ejection fraction as a marker of left ventricular function, it is important to consider the associated changes in left ventricular volumes [50]. The main ANZ carvedilol trial [45] demonstrated a 26% reduction in a combined end point of death or hospital admission after 20 months of treatment. Thus, the beneficial effect of carvedilol on left ventricular remodeling reported in the ANZ substudy [50] would be consistent with favorable effects of this agent on mortality.

These benefits of *β*-blocker treatment are neither limited to heart failure resulting from ischemic heart disease nor to treatment with carvedilol. Hall et al. [30] could demonstrate that in patients with heart failure due to both ischemic heart disease and idiopathic dilated cardiomyopathy, long-term (18 months) metoprolol treatment resulted in a significant reduction of left ventricular volumes and mass. Left ventricular shape became less spherical and assumed a more normal elliptical shape. These morphological changes were paralleled by an improvement in left ventricular ejection fraction. The studies on metoprolol [30] and carvedilol [50] both indicate that the addition of long-term *β*-blockade to background therapy with ACE-inhibitors confers additional benefit by reducing ventricular remodeling. Thus, these observations suggest that *β*-blocking agents may not simply slow remodeling, but may actually reverse it [30]. Further studies elucidating this pathophysiological context are to be awaited.

In more than 20 trials in which *β*-blocker treatment in patients with heart failure was investigated, a mean increase in left ventricular ejection fraction of 7.7% was observed [57]. This improvement in hemodynamics was independent of the underlying genesis of heart failure (IDC or ICM), the amount of left ventricular ejection fraction at baseline and the kind of *β*-blocker used (bisoprolol, bucindolol, carvedilol or metoprolol). As previously mentioned, the time course of change in ventricular function is of particular importance. Hall et al. [30] could demonstrate that at day 1 of metoprolol treatment, left ventricular ejection fraction was

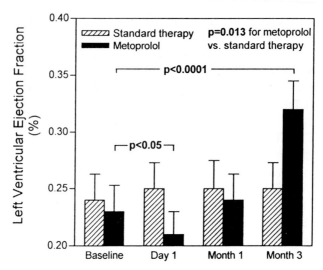

Fig. 7. Changes in left ventricular ejection fraction from baseline to day 1, month 1 and month 3 in the metoprolol and standard therapy group [from 30]

depressed but returned to baseline by month 1 and improved between months 1 and 3 (Fig. 7). By the third month of therapy there was a significant increase in left ventricular ejection fraction in the patients of the metoprolol group as compared with those in the standard therapy group. These results are consistent with the observations of Waagstein et al. [46] (see above) regarding ventricular filling pressures and cardiac index and may be an explanation for the common problem that many patients with heart failure report temporal deterioration of symptoms at the onset of β-blocker therapy. Thus, it is very important to initiate β-blocker therapy in these patients at very low doses in order to avoid decompensation of heart failure due to the pharmacological acute effects of β-blockers. Nevertheless, to achieve optimal effects of treatment, low initial doses should be titrated up to the maximum tolerated dose within several weeks.

Exercise Tolerance

The significance of exercise tolerance as a criterion for successful treatment of heart failure is controversial. Clinical trials have not sufficiently demonstrated a correlation between exercise tolerance and mortality [58]. Furthermore, it is questionable whether the tolerance of maximal exercise is important for improving quality of life, or whether the assessment of submaximal exercise tolerance (i.e., by the 6-min walk distance) is a more adequate way to determine one's ability to cope with situations in everyday life. In this context Hash and Prisant [57] compared the results of most studies on *β*-blockers in heart failure with regard to maximal and submaximal exercise tolerance. They found that *β*-blockers have a greater effect on submaximal exercise capacity than on maximal capacity. An improvement in maximal exercise capacity was observed only with metoprolol treatment, whereas carvedilol only improved submaximal exercise tolerance. The absence of improvement in maximal exercise capacity has been attributed to the attenuation of peak exercise heart rate by *β*-blockers. Bristow et al. [43] found a significant direct correlation between the reduction in maximum exercise time and reduction in peak exercise heart rate. The fact that in some studies improvement in maximal exercise can be achieved under *β*-blockade despite attenuation of maximal exercise heart rate suggests that in these patients the treatment with *β*-blockers leads to an improved cardiac contractility.

The different effects of metoprolol and carvedilol on exercise capacity might be due to the differences in *β*-adrenoceptor interaction between these two compounds. As previously described, there is a 60%–70% reduction of cardiac β_1-receptor density in patients with severe heart failure. In addition, the responsiveness of β_2-receptors is reduced by 30% due to uncoupling from the adenylyl cyclase system [26], and the *α*-subunit of the inhibitory G-protein is overexpressed [12]. Metoprolol therapy leads to a reversal of these pathological changes and to an improved response of the heart to catecholamines [59] and milrinone [60], an inhibitor of the adenosine 3',5'-monophosphate (cAMP)-phosphodiesterase (PDE III). This indicates that a blockade of cardiac *β*–adrenoceptors by metoprolol can be overcome by high levels of catecholamines, and the increased positive inotropic effect of catecholamines appears to be due to the improvements in the *β*–adrenergic system (increased receptor density and decreased levels of $G_{i\alpha}$). White et al. [61] examined the relationship between cardiac *β*-adrenoceptor density and maximal exercise capacity in 72 patients with idiopathic dilated cardiomyopathy. They observed that of all variables, maximal exercise oxygen consumption had the highest correlation with β-receptor density. In the same study, metoprolol treatment, but not carvedilol- or bucindolol treatment led to an increase in left ventricular β-receptor density. When taking into account that maximal exercise capacity is only improved by metoprolol treatment, whereas carvedilol improves submaximal exercise capacity, it can be concluded that "peripheral adaptations (i.e., by the intrinsic vasodilating effects of carvedilol) play a more important role in the ability to sustain submaximal exercise, with β-adrenergic signal transduction being more important in the cardiac response to peak exercise" [61].

Mortality

As described in the preceding chapters, β-blocker treatment in patients with heart failure improves symptoms and cardiac function. It seems likely that these beneficial effects could also prolong survival. However, this cannot be taken as proven. Milrinone, an inhibitor of phosphodiesterase (PDE III), improved symptoms and exercise capacity in patients with heart failure, but caused an increase in mortality of these patients (PROMISE trial) [62]. Recent data of the DIG study [63] demonstrated that treatment with digoxin improved symptoms and reduced hospitalization in patients with heart failure, but had no effects on survival. Thus, Lipicky and Packer [64] state that "in the area of heart failure, no surrogate end point currently exists that can be used in lieu of the direct assessment of a drug on survival, ideally in the context of a placebo-controlled trial".

The MDC trial [39] enrolled 383 patients with heart failure due to idiopathic dilated cardiomyopathy, of whom 94% were in NYHA functional class II or III. Patients were treated with either metoprolol or placebo for 18 months. Although there was no reduction of overall mortality, the combined end point of death or need for transplantation was reduced by metoprolol treatment by 34% (relative %).

The CIBIS trial [41] included mainly patients in NYHA functional class III, and half of the study population had heart failure due to ischemic heart disease. After 23 months of treatment there was no

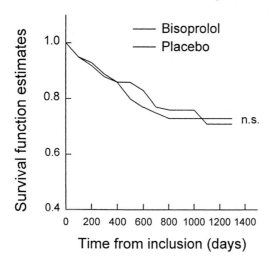

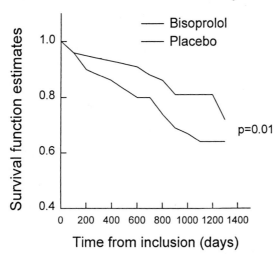

Fig. 8. Effect of bisoprolol treatment on survival in patients with heart failure with and without a history of mycardial infarction (MI) [from 41]

reduction in overall mortality. However, when looking at subgroup analysis, bisoprolol treatment significantly reduced mortality in patients without a history of myocardial infarction by 50%, whereas in patients with heart failure and a history of myocardial infarction, bisoprolol had no effect on mortality (Fig. 8). As no stratification based on etiology of heart failure was performed at randomization and thus patients did not entirely undergo coronary angiography, one has to be careful in interpreting these results.

The ANZ study on carvedilol [45] consisted exclusively of patients with mild heart failure due to ischemic heart disease. Treatment with carvedilol caused a 26% reduction of the combined end point death or hospitalization after 19 months, but no increase of overall mortality. This result may be due to the fairly good overall prognosis of patients in the study population. In the US Carvedilol Heart Failure Study Program patients were assigned to one of four treatment protocols on the basis of their exercise capacity. Thus, the US trials consisted of patients with mild [65], moderate [66, 67] and severe [68] heart failure. After 6.5 months of treatment, the overall mortality in all four protocols was reduced by 65% by treatment with carvedilol [44] (Fig. 9), independent of the underlying etiology of heart failure (IDC or ICM) and the severity of heart failure (Fig. 10). This finding led the Data and Monitoring Board to recommend termination of the study before its scheduled completion. Pfeffer and Stevenson [69] criticized that

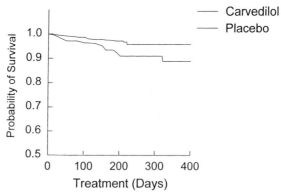

Fig. 9. The effect of carvedilol treatment on survival in patients with chronic heart failure [from 44]

Effects of Carvedilol on Mortality

1052 patients, NYHA II–IV, EF<35%, termination after 25 months

Mortality	Placebo	Carvedilol	Risk reduction
Total	7.8%	3.2%	65% (p<0.0001)
NYHA II	6.0%	2.0%	60% (p<0.05)
NYHA III–IV	11.0%	4.0%	67% (p<0.05)
IDC	6.7%	2.5%	65% (p<0.05)
ICM	9.0%	3.9%	65% (p<0.01)

Packer et al., NEJM 1996; 334:1349–1355

Fig. 10. Subgroup analysis of mortality in the US carvedilol trial [from 44]

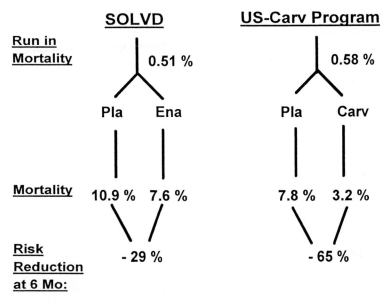

Fig. 11. Comparison of mortality and run-in mortality in the SOLVD [3] and the US carvedilol trial [44]

this was not the result of a single, definitive trial with adequate power to detect changes in mortality, and that there was a censoring of seven deaths during the run-in period. This 2-week period was designed to test the patients' ability to tolerate the drug tested. However, this 0.6% mortality rate during the run-in period of the US carvedilol trial (Fig. 11) is comparable to the mortality rate of the run-in period of the SOLVD treatment trial [3].

Cleland et al. [38] summarized the data of the four large trials on three different β-blockers (bisoprolol, carvedilol and metoprolol), with more than 2500 patients suffering from heart failure altogether. The mortality on placebo was 12.8%, falling to 8.3% on a β-blocker over a follow-up period of about 13 months, a relative risk reduction of about 37% and an absolute benefit of 45 lives saved per 1000 treated. This absolute benefit is similar to that of ACE inhibition in the SOLVD treatment trial [3], in which about 35 lives were saved per 1000 treated with enalapril at 15 months. In the SOLVD treatment trial, the 1-year mortality rate of 16% on placebo fell to 12% on enalapril. When extrapolating the 7.8% mortality rate on placebo in the US carvedilol trial to a 1-year period, the result is comparable to the mortality rate of the active treatment group of the SOLVD treatment trial. In all four trials most patients in the placebo groups received standard therapy including ACE inhibitors. Therefore the effect of β-blockers can be viewed as an additional benefit. Even if the results on mortality are not yet sufficient, the results on symptoms and hospitalization indicate a clear benefit for the patients, whose quality of life has fairly improved, besides the economic advantages of β-blocking treatment of heart failure. For these reasons, carvedilol was the first β-blocking agent to be approved for the treatment of stable chronic heart failure in the USA and Germany in 1997.

Future Studies

In order to reduce uncertainty as to the effects of β-blockers on survival, further large placebo-controlled trials are needed. These are underway with bisoprolol (CIBIS II), metoprolol (MERIT) and bucindolol (BEST). Furthermore, the COPERNICUS trial is investigating whether carvedilol improves survival compared to placebo in patients (who are in hospital) with severe heart failure. To assess whether the different pharmacological properties of metoprolol and carvedilol have different effects on survival, a comparative trial (COMET) has been initiated. The CAPRICORN trial will test whether carvedilol influences ventricular remodeling and the progress of left ventricular dysfunction to manifest heart failure in patients after myocardial infarction.

Doses

As already mentioned in the chapter "Hemodynamics", β-blockers have a potential negative inotropic effect. Thus, in patients with heart failure, it is essential to initiate treatment with β-blockers at very low doses in order to avoid decompensation. The treated patient should be in a stable condition for at least 2 weeks and should receive standard therapy consisting of diuretics, digitalis and ACE inhibitors. As patients with heart failure have a bad prognosis and tend to decompensate even at slight worsening of cardiac function, β-blockers should be regarded as additional treatment and should not replace one of the standard drugs. In the US trials even β-blockers with beneficial hemodynamic properties, such as carvedilol, showed no reduction of hospitalization in patients with severe heart failure (NYHA III–IV) [68], although in less severe cases of heart failure hospitalization was reduced. As long-term treatment with carvedilol exerted beneficial effects on survival of patients with mild, moderate or severe heart failure (Fig. 12), the temporary lack of symptomatic improvement in patients with severe symptoms does not necessarily indicate a lack of efficacy, but is rather an indicator for the biphasic character of pharmacological activity of β-blockers that was also mentioned in the chapter "Hemodynamics". As shown by the study of Hall et al. [30] (Fig. 7), a beneficial effect of β-blockers on ventricular function cannot be expected until the third month of treatment. As the hemodynamic parameters are consistent with clinical observations, during this critical period of the first 3 months a rather careful observation of the patients is indicated. Patients with severe heart failure may be admitted to hospital during this period.

Table 2 summarizes the dose pattern of β-blocker treatment of heart failure. It is highly important to initiate therapy with very low doses. According to clinical response, the dose should be doubled at 2-week intervals towards the target dose. In patients who experience worsening symptoms of chronic heart failure, the doses of ACE inhibitor or diuretic, or both, should be increased, whereas the doses of these agents should be reduced in the event of symptomatic hypotension. Figure 13 illustrates that the effects of β-blocking therapy on ejection fraction and mortality are dose-dependent. Thus, achieving the target dose is important for the therapeutical success of β-blocker treatment.

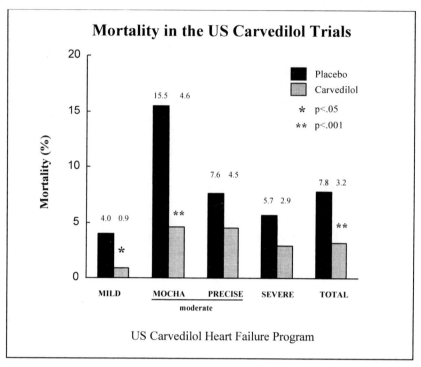

Fig. 12. Mortality in the US carvedilol trials of the US Carvedilol Failure Program

Which Patients Should Be Treated?

Patients with chronic heart failure should be in a stable condition before they are put on β-blockers. Patients with bronchial asthma should not receive β-blockers. Tachycardia can be an indicator for increased sympathetic activation. In patients with an increased heart rate at rest, β-blockers might be of special benefit as these patients profit especially from the negative inotropic effect of these compounds. In the mortality studies of β-blockade, the mean age of patients has ranged from 49 years to 67 years, whereas the mean age of chronic heart failure patients in the community is 74 years [70]. However, the US carvedilol trials suggest that the mortality benefits were similar in patients above and be-

Table 2. Dosages of *β*-blockers in heart failure

- Test dose: carvedilol (3.125 mg), metoprolol (5 mg), bisoprolol (1.25 mg) under medical supervision (2 h)
- Starting dose: carvedilol (3.125 mg b.i.d.), metoprolol (5 mg b.i.d.) bisoprolol (1.25 mg o.d.)
- Titration: doubling at 2-week intervals under medical control
- Target dose: carvedilol (2×25 mg), metoprolol (3×50 mg), bisoprolol (5 mg), or highest tolerated dose

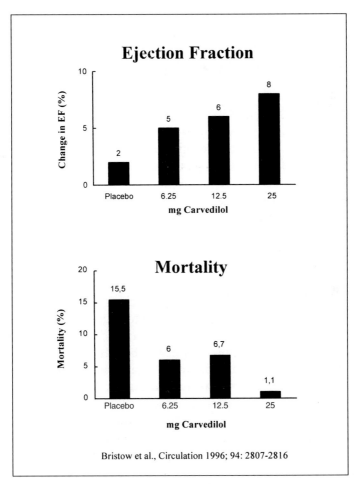

Fig. 13. Effect of various concentrations of carvedilol on left ventricular ejection fraction and mortality [from 66]

low the median age. Thus, a patients age appears to have no impact on the efficacy of β-blocking treatment of heart failure. The underlying etiology of heart failure could also be relevant. The CIBIS I trial [41] demonstrated a reduction of mortality in patients with heart failure due to idiopathic dilated cardiomyopathy by bisoprolol, whereas this agent had no effect on survival in patients with a history of myocardial infarction. Dilated cardiomyopathy, however, accounts for only a minority of patients with chronic heart failure, whereas ischemic heart disease or chronic pressure overload are responsible in most cases [71]. The ANZ study comes closest to representing this population, but in this study carvedilol only exerted benefits regarding the combined end point of death and hospitalization, whereas there was no benefit solely for overall mortality. On the other hand, the US carvedilol trials suggest that the mortality benefits are similar in patients with or without ischemic heart disease [44], while β-blockers have been shown to have important prognostic benefits in patients exhibiting chronic heart failure after myocardial infarction. Taken together, no final conclusion regarding the choice of β-blocker for a certain etiology of heart failure can be drawn from the results of the trials mentioned here. Thus, further results from future trials must be analyzed.

Summary

The treatment of heart failure with β-blockers is rational, as it is a pharmacological prevention of the deleterious effects of the elevated plasma norepinephrine levels on cardiac function that occur in patients with heart failure. Clinical trials demonstrated a beneficial effect of β-blocker treatment on symptoms, ventricular function, hospitalization and probably also on survival. Thus, β-blockers can be used in addition to standard therapy consisting of diuretics, digitalis and ACE inhibitors. However, especially in patients with severe heart failure, careful initiation and uptitration of the applied doses is of great importance. As heart failure is still a syndrome with poor prognosis, future studies will help to clarify whether β-blockers are beneficial for survival in these patients.

References

1. Smith WM (1985) Epidemiology of congestive heart failure. Am J Cardiol 55:3–8
2. The CONSENSUS Trial Study Group (1987) Effects of enalapril on mortality in severe congestive heart failure. Results of the Cooperative North Scandinavian Enalapril Survival Study (CONSENSUS). N Engl J Med 316:1429–1435
3. The SOLVD Investigators (1991) Effects of enalapril on survival in patients with reduced left ventricular ejection fractions and congestive heart failure. N Engl J Med 325:293–302
4. Australia-New Zealand Heart Failure Research Collaborative Group (1995) Effects of Carvedilol, a vasodilator-beta-blocker, in patients with congestive heart failure due to ischemic heart disease. Circulation 92:212–218
5. Waagstein F, Hjalmarson A, Varnauskas E, Wallentin I (1975) Effect of chronic beta-adrenergic receptor blockade in congestive cardiomyopathy. Br Heart J 37:1022–1036
6. Swedberg K, Hjalmarson A, Waagstein F, Wallentin I (1979) Prolongation of survival in congestive cardiomyopathy by beta-receptor blockade. Lancet 1:1374–1376
7. Swedberg K, Hjalmarson A, Waagstein F, Wallentin I (1980) Adverse effects of beta-blocker withdrawal in patients with congestive cardiomyopathy. Br Heart J 44:134–142
8. Swedberg K, Hjalmarson A, Waagstein F, Wallentin I (1980) Beneficial effects of long-term beta-blockade in congestive cardiomyopathy. Br Heart J 44:117–133
9. Cohn JN, Levine TB, Olivari MT, Gerberg V, Lura D, Francis GS, Simon AB, Rector T (1984) Plasma norepinephrine as a guide to prognosis in patients with chronic congestive heart failure. N Engl J Med 311:819–823
10. Hausdorff WP, Caron MG, Lefkowitz RJ (1990) Turning off the signal: desensitization of β–adrenergic receptor function. FASEB J 4:2881–2889
11. Bristow MR, Ginsburg R, Minobe W, et al (1982) Decreased catecholamine sensitivity and β–adrenergic receptor density in failing human hearts. N Engl J Med 307:205–211
12. Böhm M, Gierschik P, Jakobs KH, Pieske B, Schnabel P, Ungerer M, Erdmann E (1990) Increase of Giα in human hearts with dilated but not ischemic cardiomyopathy. Circulation 82:1249–1265
13. Ungerer M, Böhm M, Elce JS, Erdmann E, Lohse MJ (1993) Altered expression of β–adrenergic receptor kinase and β1-adrenergic receptors in the failing human heart. Circulation 87:454–463
14. Gage J, Rutman H, Lucido D, Le Jemtel TH (1986) Additive effects of Dobutamine and amrinone on myocardial contractility and ventricular performance in patients with severe heart failure. Circulation 74:367–373

15. Schwartz A, Lindenmayer GE, Harigaya S (1968) Respiratory control and calcium transport in heart mitochondria from the cardiomyopathic hamster. Trans N Y Acad Sci 30 (Suppl 2):951

16. Feldman MD, Alderman JD, Aroesty JM, et al (1988) Depression of systolic and diastolic myocardial reserve during atrial pacing tachycardia in patients with dilated cardiomyopathy. J Clin Invest 82:1661–1669

17. Schwinger RHG, Böhm M, Müller-Ehmsen J, et al (1993) Effect of inotropic stimulation on the negative force-frequency-relationship in the failing human heart. Circulation 88:2267–2276

18. Eichhorn EJ, Bedotto JB, Malloy CR, et al (1990) Effects of β-adrenergic receptor blockade on myocardial function and energetics in congestive heart failure. Circulation 82:473–483

19. Andersson B, Hamm C, Persson S, et al (1994) Improved exercise hemodynamic status in dilated cardiomyopathy after beta-blockade treatment. J Am Coll Cardiol 23:1397–1404

20. Ferro G, Duilio C, Spinelli L, et al (1991) Effects of beta-blockade on the relation between heart rate and ventricular diastolic perfusion time during exercise in systemic hypertension. Am J Cardiol 68:1101–1103

21. Nicholas G, Oakley C, Pouleur H, et al (1990) Xamoterol in severe heart failure. Lancet 336:1–6

22. Gilbert EM, Anderson JL, Deitchman D, et al (1990) Long-term beta-blocker vasodilator therapy improves cardiac function in idiopathic dilated cardiomyopathy: a double-blind, randomized study of bucindolol versus placebo. Am J Med 88:223–229

23. Gilbert EM, Abraham WT, Olsen S, et al (1996) Comparative hemodynamic, left ventricular functional and antiadrenergic effects of chronic treatment with metoprolol versus carvedilol in the failing heart. Circulation 94:2817–2825

24. Imperato-McGinley J, Gautier T, Ehlers K, et al (1987) Reversibility of catecholamine-induced dilated cardiomyopathy in a child with pheochromocytoma. N Engl J Med 316:793–797

25. Cruickshank JM, Neil-Dwyer G, Degaute JP, et al (1987) Reduction of stress/catecholamine-induced cardiac necrosis by beta1-selective blockade. Lancet 1:585–589

26. Gilbert EM, Olsen SL, Renlund DG, Bristow MR (1993) Beta-adrenergic receptor regulation and left ventricular function in idiopathic dilated cardiomyopathy. Am J Cardiol 71:23C–29C

27. Sigmund M, Jakob H, Becker H (1996) Effects of metoprolol on myocardial β-adrenoceptors and Giα-proteins in patients with congestive heart failure. Eur J Clin Pharmacol 51:127–132

28. Yoshikawa T, Port JD, Asaro K, et al (1996) Cardiac adrenergic receptor effects of carvedilol. Eur Heart J 17(Suppl. B):8–16

29. Whyte K, Jones CR, Howie CA, et al (1987) Haemodynamic metabolic and lymphocyte beta2-adrenoceptor changes following chronic beta-adrenoceptor antagonism. Eur J Clin Pharmacol 32:237–243

30. Hall SA, Cigarroa CG, Marcoux L, et al (1995) Time course of improvement in left ventricular function, mass and geometry in patients with congestive heart failure treated with beta-adrenergic blockade. J Am Coll Cardiol 25:1154–6131

31. Kukin ML, Kalman J, Mannino M, et al (1996) Combined alpha-betablockade (doxazosin and metoprolol) compared with beta-blockade alone in chronic congestive heart failure. Am J Cardiol 77:486–491

32. Yue TL, Cheng H-J, Lysko PG, et al (1992) Carvedilol, a new vasodilator and beta-adrenoceptor antagonist, is an antioxidant and free radical scavenger. J Pharmacol Exp Ther 263:92–98

33. Yue T-L, Liu T, Feuerstein G (1992) Carvedilol, a new vasodilator and beta-adrenoceptor antagonist, inhibits oxygen radical mediated lipid peroxidation in swine ventricular membranes. Pharmacol Communications 1:27–35

34. Bolli R (1990) Mechanisms of myocardial stunning. Circulation 82:723–738

35. Belch JJF, Bridges AB, Scott N, Chopra M (1991) Oxygen free radicals in congestive heart failure. Br Heart J 65:245–248

36. Sung C-P, Arleth AJ, Ohlstein EH (1993) Carvedilol inhibits vascular smooth muscle cell proliferation. J Cardiovasc Pharmacol 21:221–227

37. Ohlstein EH, Douglas SA, Sung C-P, et al (1993) Carvedilol, a cardiovascular drug, prevents vascular smooth muscle cell proliferation, migration and neointimal formation following vascular injury. Proc Natl Acad Sci U S A 90:6189–6193

38. Cleland JGF, Bristow MR, Erdmann E, Remme WJ, Swedberg K, Waagstein F (1996) Beta-blocking agents in heart failure – should they be used and how? Eur Heart J 17:1629–1639

39. Waagstein F, Bristow MR, Swedberg K, et al (1993) Beneficial effects of metoprolol in idiopathic dilated cardiomyopathy. Lancet 342:1441–1446

40. Fisher ML, Gottlieb SS, Plotnick G, et al (1994) Beneficial effects of metoprolol in heart failure associated with coronary artery disease: a randomized trial. J Am Coll Cardiol 23:943–950

41. CIBIS Investigators and Committees (1994) A randomized trial of *β*-blockade in heart failure. The Cardiac Insufficiency Bisoprolol Study (CIBIS). Circulation 90:1765–1773

42. Woodley SL, Gilbert EM, Anderson JL, et al (1991) *β*-blockade with bucindolol in heart failure caused by ischemic versus idiopathic dilated cardiomyopathy. Circulation 84:2426–2441

43. Bristow MR, O'Connel JB, Gilbert EM, et al (1994) Dose-response of chronic *β*-blocker treatment in heart failure from either idiopathic dilated or ischemic cardiomyopathy. Circulation 89:1632–1642

44. Packer M, Bristow MR, Cohn JN, et al. for the US carvedilol study group (1996) The effect of carvedilol on morbidity and mortality in patients with chronic heart failure. N Engl J Med 334:1349–1355

45. Australia-New Zealand Heart Failure Research Collaborative Group (1997) Randomized, placebo-controlled trial of carvedilol in patients with congestive heart failure due to ischemic heart disease. Lancet 349:375–380

46. Waagstein F, Caidahl K, Wallentin I, et al (1989) Long-term beta-blockade in dilated cardiomyopathy: effects of short- and long-term metoprolol treatment followed by withdrawal and readministration of metoprolol. Circulation 80:551–563

47. Lahiri A, Rodrigues EA, Al-Khawaja I, et al (1987) Effect of a new vasodilating beta-blocking drug, carvedilol, on left ventricular function in stable angina-pectoris. Am J Cardiol 59:769–774

48. Awan NA, Needham KE, Evenson MK, et al (1981) Therapeutic application of prazosin in chronic refractory congestive heart failure: tolerance and "tachyphylaxis" in perspective. Am J Med 71:153–160

49. Metra M, Nardi M, Giubbini R (1994) Effects of short- and long-term carvedilol administration on rest and exercise hemodynamic variables, exercise capacity and clinical conditions in patients with idiopathic dilated cardiomyopathy. J Am Coll Cardiol 24:1678–1687

50. Doughty RN, Whalley GA, Gamble G, et al. on behalf of the Australia-New Zealand Heart Failure Research Collaborative Group (1997) Left ventricular remodeling with carvedilol in patients with congestive heart failure due to ischemic heart disease. J Am Coll Cardiol 29:1060–1066

51. Gaudron P, Eilles C, Kugler I, Ertl G (1993) Progressive left ventricular dysfunction and remodeling after myocardial infarction. Potential mechanisms and early predictors. Circulation 87:755–763

52. Hammermeister KE, De Rouen TA, Dodge HAT (1979) Variables predictive of survival in patients with coronary disease: selection by univariate and multivariate analyses from the clinical, electrocardiographic, exercise, arteriographic and quantitative angiographic evaluations. Circulation 59:421–430

53. White HD, Norris RM, Brown MA, Brandt PWT, Whitlock RML, Wild CJ (1987) Left ventricular end-systolic volume as the major determinant of survival after recovery from myocardial infarction. Circulation 76:44–51

54. Sharpe N, Murphy J, Smith H, Hannan S (1988) Treatment of patients with symptomless left ventricular dysfunction after myocardial infarction. Lancet:255–259

55. Sutton MSJ, Pfeffer MA, Plappert T, et al (1994) Quantitative two-dimensional echocardiographic measurements are major predictors of adverse cardiovascular events after acute myocardial infarction. Circulation 89:68–75

56. Cohn JN (1994) Vasodilators in heart failure: conclusions from V-HeFT II and rationale for V-HeFT III. Drugs 47(Suppl 4):47–58

57. Hash TW, Prisant LM (1997) β–blocker use in systolic heart failure and dilated cardiomyopathy. J Am Coll Cardiol 37:7–19

58. Swedberg K (1994) Exercise testing in heart failure: a critical review. Drugs 47(Suppl 4):14–24
59. Heilbrunn SM, Shah P, Bristow MR, et al (1989) Increased *β*–receptor density and improved hemodynamic response to catecholamine stimulation during long-term metoprolol therapy in heart failure from dilated cardiomyopathy. Circulation 79:483–490
60. Böhm M, Deutsch HJ, Hartmann D, La Rosée K, Stäblein A (1997) Improvement of postreceptor events by metoprolol treatment in patients with chronic heart failure. J Am Coll Cardiol 30:992–996
61. White M, Yanowitz F, Gilbert EM, et al (1995) Role of *β*–adrenergic receptor downregulation in the peak exercise response in patients with heart failure due to idiopathic dilative cardiomyopathy. Am J Cardiol 76:1271–1276
62. Packer M, Arver JR, Rodeheffer RJ, et al. for the PROMISE Study Research Group (1991) Effect of oral milrinone on mortality in severe chronic heart failure. N Engl J Med 325:1468–1475
63. The Digitalis Investigation Group (DIG) (1997) The effect of digoxin on mortality and morbidity in patients with heart failure. N Engl J Med 336:525–533
64. Lipicky RJ, Packer M (1993) Role of surrogate end points in the evaluation of drugs for heart failure. J Am Coll Cardiol 22(Suppl A):179A–184A
65. Colucci WS, Packer M, Bristow MR, et al (1996) Carvedilol inhibits clinical progression in patients with mild symptoms of heart failure. Circulation 94:2800–2806
66. Bristow MR, Gilbert EM, Abraham WT, Adams KF, Fowler MB, Hershberger RE, Kubo SH, Narahara KA, Ingersoll H, Krueger S, Young S, Shusterman N (1996) Carvedilol produces dose-related improvements in left ventricular function and survival in subjects with chronic heart failure. MOCHA Investigators [comment]. Circulation 94:2807–2816
67. Packer M, Colucci WS, Sackner-Bernstein JD, Liang CS et al. for the PRECISE Study Group (1996) Double-blind, placebo controlled study of the effects of carvedilol in patients with moderate to severe heart failure: the PRECISE trial. Circulation 94:2793–2799
68. Cohn J, Fowler MB, Bristow MR, et al (1997) Safety and efficacy of carvedilol in severe chronic heart failure. J Card Failure 3:173–179
69. Pfeffer MA, Stevenson LW (1996) *β*–adrenergic blockers and survival in heart failure. N Engl J Med 334:1396–1397
70. Parmershwar J, Shackel MM, Richardson A, Poole-Wilson PA, Sutton GC (1992) Prevalence of heart failure in three general practices in northwest London. Br J Gen Pract 42:287–289
71. Sutton GC (1990) Epidemiologic aspects of heart failure. Am Heart J 120:1538–1540
72. Marwood JF, Stokes GS (1986) Studies on the vasodilator actions of bucindolol in the rat. Clin Exp Pharmacol Physiol 13:59–68

CHAPTER 11

Heart Failure:
Treatment with β-Adrenoceptor Antagonists

PHILIP A. POOLE-WILSON

Introduction

Advances in the understanding of the underlying pathophysiology of heart failure, the availability of heart transplantation and the introduction of new drugs have transformed the treatment of heart failure. In the early part of this century the treatment of heart failure was bed-rest, diet, control of fluid intake and a variety of unpleasant manoeuvres aimed at the reduction of fluid accumulation. Substantial controversy surrounded the use of digoxin whose properties had so clearly been described by Withering in 1785 [1]. Benefit from digoxin accrued to patients with the combination of heart failure and atrial fibrillation because control of the heart rate was achieved. Benefit for patients with heart failure in sinus rhythm was less certain at that time, although there was a strong belief that a positive inotropic agent should be advantageous to patients. The treatment of heart failure was transformed by the introduction of diuretics and in particular by the use of thiazide diuretics [2]. Later a series of trials demonstrated the benefit of adding an angiotensin converting enzyme (ACE) inhibitor to the use of a diuretic in heart failure [3–5]. In the 1980s the value of using digoxin in patients with heart failure who were in sinus rhythm and who had been optimally treated with diuretics was challenged again [6–8]. A recent large trial has provided only limited evidence of clinical efficacy and no benefit in terms of mortality [9].

Thus the standard treatment for heart failure (Table 1) is a diuretic and ACE inhibitor with or without digoxin. In selected patients an argument can be made for the addition of aspirin, warfarin or an anti-arrhythmic agent. Other drugs are used less often.

Table 1. Options in the treatment of heart failure

1. Drugs	Diuretics	Loop, thiazide, K$^+$ sparing, spironolactaone or combination
	ACE inhibitors	
	Vasodilators	Nitrates, hydralazine
	Positive inotropes	Digoxin, IV intermittent inotrope
	Anticoagulants, β-blockers, calcium antagonists, antiarrhythmics or angiotensin II receptor inhibitors	

2. Surgery, CABG or valve surgery
3. Implantable cardioverter-defibrillator – ICD, pacing
4. Haemofiltration, peritoneal dialysis or haemodialysis
5. Aortic balloon pump, ventricular assist devices cardiomyoplasty, volume reduction, transplantation

This description of the standard treatment for heart failure (Table 1) has now been challenged by the proposition that chronic β-adrenergic receptor blockade (with a β-blocker) should be added to the combination of a diuretic and an ACE inhibitor in the majority of patients with heart failure. The issues facing the clinician are whether the evidence is sufficiently strong to support such a view, how patients should be selected for treatment with a β-blocker and how treatment with a β-blocker should be initiated.

Pathophysiology of Heart Failure

There have been numerous attempts to define the clinical entity of heart failure. None are entirely satisfactory and most emphasise one or other aspect of the syndrome such as the haemodynamics, exercise capacity or metabolism considered in terms of oxygen consumption. Heart failure is a clinical syndrome and for practical purposes is "a clinical syndrome caused by an abnormality of the heart and recognised by a characteristic pattern of haemodynamic, renal, neural and hormonal responses" [10]. Most of the common clinical signs of chronic heart failure are related to sodium and water retention that is a consequence of reduced renal excretion [11, 12]. The commonest symptoms are fatigue and breathlessness. The origins of these symptoms are complex and not simply related to central haemodynamics or the cardiac output but rather to signals emanating from skeletal muscle and the peripheral circulation [13–17].

There are many causes for heart failure and many different clinical presentations. In the past phrases such as right and left, high and low output, forward and backward have been popular [10]. Most of these terms relate to redundant or incorrect concepts. It is useful both clinically and conceptually to distinguish between acute and chronic heart failure. The distinction between systolic and diastolic heart failure is also important because of the confusion that this distinction can promulgate. Systolic heart failure is a term used when the ventricle is enlarged subsequent to damage caused either by an event consequent upon coronary artery disease or as part of a cardiomyopathy. Diastolic heart failure is a term used when symptoms attributable the heart occur in the presence of a normal sized heart in end-diastole. The diagnosis is often made after the measurement of a normal ejection fraction in the presence of signs or symptoms of heart failure. Diastolic heart failure is particularly common in the elderly, in the presence of long-standing coronary heart disease, hypertension or myocardial hypertrophy. It is notoriously difficult to treat. Although this entity is called diastolic heart failure the symptoms and signs may be related in large part but not directly to systolic malfunction as well as diastolic malfunction of the heart as a pump.

In the 1960s it was widely held that the major and underlying abnormality in heart failure was an inability of the heart to emit blood and that a positive inotropic drug would, therefore, bring about substantial benefit as a consequence of greater contraction of the muscle of the heart. Clinical studies have demonstrated otherwise. Almost all positive inotropic drugs of whatever class appear to hasten death. The one exception may be transient use of inotropic agents to resolve acute episodes of heart failure. The harmful effect is related not just to an increased tendency for arrhythmias but to a progressive worsening of heart failure probably the result of an increased rate of loss of cells (apoptosis). The only drug with a positive inotropic effect, that might improve symptoms (although to a minor degree) but has a neutral effect on mortality, is digoxin [9].

In the 1970s and 1980s emphasis moved to the identification and characterisation of the neuroendocrine response to heart fail-

Table 2. Hormonal mediators in heart failure

Constrictors	Dilators	Growth factors
Noradrenaline	ANP	Insulin
Renin/angiotensin II	Prostaglandin E2	TNF alpha
Vasopressin	& metabolites	Growth hormone
NPY	EDRF	Angiotensin II
Endothelin	Dopamine	Catecholamines
	CGRP	NO
		Cytokines
		Oxygen radicals

ure (Table 2) and the possible advantageous role of drugs which block some of these responses. Of particular note were activation of the sympathetic system and the renin-angiotensin system. The renin-angiotensin system is not activated early in heart failure [18, 19] unlike the sympathetic system and atrial and brain natriuretic peptides (ANF and BNP). A major stimulus to the activation of the renin-angiotensin system is the use of diuretics to control fluid volumes [12, 18]. Indeed the use of ACE inhibitors in heart failure can to a large extent be considered as a counter to this undesirable side-effect of diuretics.

Numerous endocrine abnormalities have been reported in heart failure (Table 2) and this lead to the hormonal hypothesis of heart failure according to which the progression of heart failure was attributable to the consequences of elevation of these hormones. If such a hypothesis were correct then inhibition should be beneficial. This was the initial scientific basis for the use of angiotensin converting enzyme inhibitors.

In recent years the understanding of heart failure has become more complex. Many symptoms are linked not to haemodynamics or to hormone activation but to the body response to heart failure and in particular alterations in the peripheral circulation and skeletal muscle [15–17]. The progressive malfunction of the heart itself may be attributable either to further manifestations of coronary artery disease or to processes that bring about an increase in the loss of myocytes. Cardiac myocytes are lost naturally during the ageing process and mitosis of this cell type is believed to cease soon after birth. The natural loss is aggravated by ischaemia, metabolic stress (including that brought about by positive inotropic agents), hypertension or myocardial hypertrophy. Myocytes may die either by necrosis or apoptosis [21, 21]. The residual myocardium will hypertrophy and the shape of the ventricle alter (remodelling). There is a possibility that cell division could occur by a process other than mitosis since many cells (perhaps 15%) in the adult human myocardium are binucleate or exhibit polyploidy having double the normal content of DNA. Stimulation of the biochemical pathways concerned with the loss of cells (apoptosis) is almost certainly linked to the activation of cytokines systems (Table 2) [22, 23]. The inhibition of these cytokine systems is a new direction for the treatment of heart failure.

Mechanisms of Action of β-Blockers in Heart Failure

A possible treatment for heart failure is inhibition of the sympathetic system by use of a β-blocker (Table 3). Some actions and clinical applications of β-blockers are clearly described and not contentious. These drugs are advantageous in the treatment of angina pectoris and hypertension. In addition β-blockers may reduce hypertrophy in hypertension and minimise ischaemia. In clinical situations where ventricular filling is slow and tachycardia reduces the total proportion of diastolic time, β-blockers can increase cardiac output. That is particularly evident in patients with tachycardia and mitral stenosis or in patients (often elderly) with

Table 3. Mode of action of β-blockers in heart failure

Certain
1. Anti-ischaemic effect
2. Reduction of blood pressure (hypotensive effect)
3. Improved ventricular filling when tachycardia exists with functional mitral regurgtation

Possible
4. Anti-arrhythmic effect
5. Improved diastolic function
6. Reduced oxygen consumption
7. Reduced damage from raised plasma catecholamines

heart failure, tachycardia, small hearts and a degree of functional mitral regurgitation. The use of β-blockers in patients with either of these conditions is well established and benefit in the presence of a mild degree of heart failure would be anticipated.

Other possible mechanisms of benefit are more controversial. Beta-blockers have an anti-arrhythmic action, which is in addition to any impact on myocardial ischaemia. Abnormal rhythms, particularly arrhythmias caused by a triggered mechanism as opposed to re-entry mechanisms, are common in patients with heart failure. Beta-blockers in general reduce myocardial oxygen consumption. Many mechanisms contribute to this effect which may be advantageous to myocytes already subject to multiple stimulatory stresses. Myocardial oxygen consumption may be diminished due partly to altered timing and more co-ordinated ventricular filling and partly to an anti-ischaemic effect. Increase in the total time in diastole per unit of time will increase coronary flow to the left ventricle, since flow to the left ventricle occurs predominantly in diastole. Catecholamines in high concentrations have been known for many years to have a direct toxic effect on the myocardium. This is evident in phaeochromacytoma and in many experimental models. Were such a mechanism to contribute to the progression of heart failure in humans then this would be a further mechanism for the putative advantageous effects of β-blockers.

Some β-blockers, carvedilol for example, have additional properties to β-blockade. Carvedilol exhibits a_1-adrenergic blockade, is an anti-oxidant and prevents smooth cell proliferation by mechanism other than β-blockade. Bucindolol is a direct vasodilator. Carvedilol and bucindolol are non-selective β-blockers exhibiting β_2 adrenoceptor antagonism whereas metoprolol and bisoprolol are β_1 selective. The extent to which these mechanisms could be or are advantageous in preventing the progression of heart failure by counteracting apoptosis or by any other mechanism is at present unknown.

Cellular Role of Catecholamines

The effect of adrenoceptor antagonists within the cardiac myocyte is clearly described. Calcium influx is increased. Phospholamban is phosphorylated and as a consequence the uptake of calcium into the sarcoplasmic reticulum is increased. Phosphorylation of the contractile proteins diminishes the calcium sensitivity of the contractile proteins. The first two mechanisms bring about increased contractility and an increased rate of relaxation, whereas the latter might be anticipated to diminish contractility. The first two mechanisms dominate.

In the human heart there are substantial numbers of β-receptors. Most β_2 receptors are on the vasculature but unlike animal models the cardiac myocyte has a substantial number of β_2 receptors, the ratio of β_1 to β_2 receptors being 80:20. Again unlike animal models, in the human cardiac myocyte there are few spare receptors so that the number of receptors relates almost directly to the functional consequences of activation. The proportion of receptors, which are on the vasculature rather than on the cardiac myocyte itself, is unknown in many studies. Single myocytes from the same heart can vary in the proportion of β_1 to β_2 receptors, which is present [24].

In heart failure the plasma level of noradrenaline is increased [25, 26] where as adrenaline is only increased in severe heart failure [11]. Sympathetic nerve traffic is increased [27]. For any level of exercise plasma noradrenaline is higher in heart failure although the maximum concentration achieved at peak exercise is greater in normal persons in whom the peak exercise level is also much greater [25, 26]. The urinary excretion of catecholamines is increased in heart failure. Within the myocardium there is no increase in catecholamines and often a reduction [28, 29]. The distribution of catecholamines in the heart is heterogeneous [30]. There is a net loss of catecholamines from the heart. Abnormalities of metabolism have been reported [31] in addition to altered re-uptake from the neuronal cleft [32] and increased spill over [33, 34]. Overall sympathetic activity is activated early in heart failure.

Down regulation of β_1 receptors was reported many years ago [35]. β_2 receptors are in general not down regulated but are uncoupled. The mechanisms of down regulation and desensitisation are many and complex [36]. In the human heart because of the lack of spare receptors the reduction in β_1 receptors goes along with a reduction in the contractile response to adrenoceptor ago-

Table 4. Objectives of treatment in chronic heart failure

1. Prevention	• Myocardial damage	• Occurrence
		• Progression of damage
		• Further damaging episodes
	• Reoccurrence	• Symptoms
		• Fluid accumulation
		• Hospitalisaiton
2. **Relief of symptoms and signs**		
	• Eliminate oedema and fluid retention	
	• Increase exercise capacity	
	• Reduce fatigue and breathlessness	
3. **Prognosis**	Reduce mortality	

nists. Inhibition of β-receptors in heart failure would be expected to and does bring about an initial negative inotropic effect. The receptors can be upregulated after long term treatment with β-adrenoceptor blockers. A greater effect might be anticipated from a non-selective β-blocker although the major part of the inotropic effect of activation of the sympathetic activity in heart failure is due to β_1 receptors because of the increase in the plasma concentration of noradrenaline rather than adrenaline. Noradrenaline is the hormone that is the principal activator of β_1 receptors.

Objectives in the Treatment of Heart Failure

The objectives of heart failure are three fold (Table 4). The first is to prevent the occurrence of the initiating causes of heart failure. The second is to improve the symptoms and quality of life of the patients. The third is to reduce mortality. Any new drug in the treatment of heart failure must be judged by these three criteria.

Outcome with the Use of β-Blockers in Heart Failure

In the last few decades it has been conventional to regard heart failure as a contra-indication to the use of a β-blocker. There is certainly strong clinical evidence that under certain circumstances β-blockers can worsen heart failure and many data sheets warn of this side-effect of β-blockade. As long ago as 1975 [37] work was undertaken to investigate the possibility that β-blockers might be advantageous in heart failure for the reasons described above (Table 5). This lead to a large number of studies many of which would not fulfil the criteria for modern clinical trials; these studies often were not randomised studies or were not blinded [38–49]. However, a few early randomised placebo controlled and blinded studies (Table 5) did suggest some advantage from β-blockade in heart failure but these studies in general were small and many suggestions were put forward to discount the claim of benefit. In recent years several larger and well conducted studies have been published [50–60] which have radically altered the perception with regard to the clinical use of β-blockers in heart failure (Table 6).

There are several findings consistent across all studies. Beta-blockers not unexpectedly reduce heart rate and result in an increase in the ejection fraction. At first sight it might be thought that these two effects were related. If the heart rate falls and the cardiac output at rest is to be maintained, then it is inevitable that there is an increase in ejection fraction. Since the filling time of the left ventricle is increased it might be anticipated that the left ventricular end-diastolic volume would increase. However recent work indicates that the increase in ejection fraction occurs in the presence of a decrease in the end diastolic volume of the ventricle and not an increase [59, 60]. That finding would argue that the change in ejection fraction is not solely related to an alteration in the heart rate but is a consequence, to some degree, of myocardial remodelling in the ventricle. The remodelling could nevertheless be a long-term consequence of the alteration in heart rate. It must also be noted that a change in the ejection fraction or heart rate is not a major objective of the treatment of heart failure. There is no simple relation between ejection fraction and symptoms in patients with heart failure, although a change of ejection fraction might be a surrogate of symptomatic benefit. In the largest single study of carvedilol the increase of ejection fraction was not associated with any change in symptoms [59, 60].

Table 5. β-Blockers for heart failure – early studies

Author	Date	Design	n	Duration [months]	Symptom	Haemod.	Exercise	Comment
Waagstein [38]	1975	O, U	7	5	Benefit	Benefit	Benefit	EF increased
Swedberg [39]	1980	O, U	28	23	Benefit	Benefit		EF increased
Heilbrunn [40]	1989	O, U	14	6	Benefit			EF increased
Nemanich [41]	1990	O, U	10	2			Benefit	EF increased
Andersson [42]	1991	O, U	21	14	Benefit	Benefit	Benefit	EF increased
Ikram [43]	1981	B, C	15	1			Reduced	LV enlarged
Currie [44]	1984	B, C	10	1	Unaltered	CI reduced		
Leung [15]	1990	B, C	12	2	Benefit	Unaltered	Benefit	
Engelmeier [46]	1985	B, R	37	12	Benefit		Benefit	EF increased
Anderson [47]	1985	B, R	50	19	Benefit		Benefit	
German/Austr. [48]	1988	B, R	329	3	Benefit		Benefit	
Xamoterol [49]	1990	B, R	616	3	Benefit		Unaltered	Increased mortality

O = open, U = uncontrolled, R = randomised, B = blind, C = crossover.

Table 6. Carvedilol β-Blockers for heart failure – recent trials

Author	n	Duration and type	EF	NYHA	Exercise	Hospital-isation	Mor-tality	Combined endpoint	% excluded
MDC, 1993 [50]	383	12 m R,D	+	+	+ at 12 m	+	=	NA	4.4
CIBIS, 1994 [51]	641	1.9 y D	NA	+	NA	+	=	NA	NR
Metra, 1994 [52]	40	4 m D	+	+	+	NA	NA	NA	0
Olsen, 1995 [53]	60	3 m D	+	+	=	NA	NA	NA	0
Krum, 1995 [54]	56	14 w R,D	+	+	+	NA	=	+	12.5
MOCHA, 1996 [55]	345	6 m R,D	+	=	=	+	+	+	8
Colucci, 1996 [56]	366	12 m R,D	+	+	=	=	=	+	6
PRECISE, 1996 [57]	278	6 m R,D	+	+	=	=	=	+	8
Cohn, 1997 58]	105	6 m R,D	+	=	=	=	=	=	10
ANZ study, 1997 [59]	415	6–19 m R,D	+	=	=	=	=	+	6

R = run-in period, *D* = double-blind and randomised, *NA* = not available, *NR* = not relevant.
Packer et al. N Engl J Med 1996; 334:1349–1355 [60].

The results of the effects of β-blockade on clinical measures of efficacy have been variable. These measures have included quality of life, symptoms, exercise capacity, hospital admissions and physician attendances (Table 6). The results from exercise studies have been particularly disappointing. It is probable that β-blockers do limit the maximum ability to exercise but it is becoming increasingly clear that the maximum ability to exercise is not a good surrogate of the quality of life in heart failure. Other evidence has suggested that an increase in the ability to exercise at a less than maximum workload is increased with a β-blocker. However the inconsistency of the data is concerning. The largest study undertaken failed to show any benefit in terms of any known outcome measure for symptoms, with the possible exception of hospitalisation [59, 60].

Interest in the use of β-blockade in heart failure has increased very substantially because of recent mortality studies and notably the study report of the four carvedilol trials (Tables 7 and 8) [61]. There have been four recent meta-analyses of mortality with β-blockers [62–66]. All of these have indicated a favourable effect on mortality with a reduction of the order of 25%. The total number of patients included in these analyses is about 3000 of whom half have participated in trials with carvedilol. The total number of deaths is about 300. These figures are too small to allow for any meaningful sub-analyses. Where that has been attempted there has not been evidence of heterogeneity or any benefit limited solely to one β-blocker or any single characteristic of this group of drugs.

Table 7. Carvedilol trials in heart failure

	Placebo	Carvedilol	RR (95% Ci)	P
n	398	696		
Total mortality	31	22	0.41 (0.24–0.69)	0.001
Hospitalisation	78	98	0.72 (0.55–0.94)	0.02
But including deaths (D) & worsening heart failure (W) in *run in period*				
Total mortality & D	31	29	0.53 (0.33–0.87)	0.02
Total mortality & D & W	31	46	0.85 (0.55–1.32)	ns
Hospitalisation & W	78	115	0.84 (0.67–1.13)	ns

Packer et al. N Engl J Med 1996; 334:1349–1355 [61].

Table 8. Carvedilol trials in heart failure

Carvedilol upto 50 mg bd, 1094 patients (placebo 398, carvedilol 696)
58 years, median follow-up 6.5 months, EF<0.35, actual EF 0.23
On diuretics, digoxin and ACE inhibitors, 3% in NYHA IV
"nonischemic dilated cardiomyopathy" in 52%

Total mortality 31/398 placebo, 22/696 carvedilol.
RR 0.41 (95% CI 0.24–0.69), P<0.00

Limitations:

53 deaths, short follow-up, 7 deaths in 17 worsening heart failure in run-in
Four trials not one trial
Safety study not mortality study

Packer et al. N Engl J Med 1996; 334:1349–1355 [61].

Table 9. Xamoterol in severe heart failure

516 patients randomised toxamoterol (200 mg bd) or placebo

Symptoms and exercise capacity unchanged
Heart rate and systolic blood pressure reduced

	Xamoterol	Placebo	
n	327	150	
Total withdrawals (%)	67 (19%)	19 (12%)	
% of withdrawals	73%	62%	
Due to cardiovascular changes			
Total deaths (%)	32 (9.1%)	6 (3.7%)	p=0.02

From Lancet 1990; 336:1–6 [49].

There is a major flaw in all three meta-analyses. It is a well established requirement of a meta-analysis that all studies are included. One study has not been included in any of these three
meta-analyses namely the study with xamoterol (Table 9) [49].
That is of particular concern because it is only this study which
reported a negative result on mortality. The trial was undertaken
in patients with severe heart failure. Patients were started on the
drug without a test dose or test run-in period nor was there uptitration of the drug. The trial was stopped because of an increase
in mortality (32/327, 9.1% on xamoterol versus 6/150, 3.7% on

placebo, $P < 0.02$). There has not been a paper on the nature of the deaths in this study. It might be argued that the increase of death was due to arrhythmias caused by a drug with intrinsic sympathomimetic effects. Alternatively the result was the true effect of initiating a full dose of a β-blocker in severely sick patients with heart failure. The omission of the study from the meta-analysis might be claimed to be reasonable and appropriate because this drug does possess different properties to the other β-blockers. Such an argument, however, smacks of trial selection and bias, since the one trial excluded had an unfavourable result and there exists a plausible scientific basis for the result, namely the use of a β-blocker in patients with severe heart failure. If this trial is added to a simple meta-analysis of the major studies then the overall results are not significant (Table 10).

The major evidence for an effect on mortality arises from the four trials undertaken in the United States with carvedilol (Tables 7 and 8) [61]. That data has important limitations. The studies were over a short period of 6 months, the studies were different in design and the overall number of events was only 53. This number of events is very much smaller than the calculated numbers required to demonstrate significance in the current large trials being undertaken. A period of follow-up as short as six months is not generally accepted as appropriate for mortality trials in patients with mild or moderate heart failure. Indeed if that were the criteria for the demonstration of efficacy then several other drugs might have claimed to have benefit but for the fact that the drugs were studied over longer periods of time and shown to be harmful.

A further major criticism of the carvedilol trials is that some patients deteriorated and were withdrawn or hospitalised during the run-in period. That is the analysis was not on the basis of intention to treat all patients but only to treat those patients who were not adversely affected in the initial test period. This design biases the trial in favour of the drug and underestimates the adverse effects which might occur if the drug were used widely and indiscriminately. If a worst case scenario is adopted for those patients and they are included in the intention to treat analysis then the overall finding of a reduction of mortality no longer pertains.

Table 10. β-blockade for heart failure and mortality – large randomised trials

	Mean follow-up (months)	Placebo deaths	%	Abs. risk reduction (%)	Relative risk (95% CI)	No. to treat to save one	P
Xamoterol	4.25	6/164	3.7	+5.4	2.7 (1.17–6.3)	18 for harm	0.02
MDC (metoprolol)	15	19/189	10.1	+1.8	1.19 (0.67–2.10)	54 for harm	ns
CIBIS (bisoprolol)	21	67/321	20.9	4.3	0.79 (0.57–1.10)	23	ns
ANZ (carvedilol)	18	26/208	12.5	2.8	0.77 (0.45–1.34)	35	ns
US trials (carvedilol)	6.5	31/398	7.8	4.6	0.35 (0.24–0.69)	21	0.001
Total		149/1280	11.6%	3.2%	OR=0.81 (0.63–1.03)	27	ns
Excluding xamoterol		143/1116	12.8%	4.5%	OR=0.71 (0.54–0.92)	22	0.01

Table 11. β-blocker trials in heart failure in progress

CIBIS 2	Cardiac insufficiency with bisoprolol study Bisoprolol vs placebo. 2500 patients. NYHA II–IV. Follow-up >3 y All cause mortality
BEST	β-blocker evaluation survival trial Bucindolol vs placebo. 2800 patients. NYHA II–IV. Non run-in period. Follow-up >18 m. All cause mortality
MERIT	Metoprolol trial Metoprolol vs placebo. 3400 patients. NYHA II–IV. No run-in period. Follow-up >3 y. All cause mortality
COMET	Carvedilol or metroprolol – european trial Carvedilol vs metoprolol. 2800 patients. NYHA II–IV. Followed until 750 fatal events with no run-in period. All cause mortality
COPERNICUS	Carvedilol vs placebo 1800 patients. NYHA III–IV. Follow-up >18 m. All cause mortality

To resolve the issues relating to the use of β-blockers in heart failure large mortality studies are needed. Five such studies are currently underway (Table 11) and their results will be reported in the next few years. Many will wonder how strong claims for the efficacy of β-blockade in terms of mortality and morbidity established by current results are compatible with the belief that it is necessary and ethically appropriate to continue with trials involving 13,300 patients (cf 3000 patients in published trials at present) over periods of at least 18 months. If the medical profession is to embrace evidence based medicine then interpretation of current data should not be exaggerated in favour of new drugs. Being an accurate prophet has some merit and much appeal but prophecy deserves little credit if large numbers of patients are needlessly put at risk. The risk is probably small in those with mild heart failure for reasons to be discussed. In severe heart failure that is not true and β-blockade should in the view of this author be used cautiously in those with more than mild heart failure.

Benefit in Sub-sets of Patients

Many cardiologists would be surprised if β-blockers were advantageous for all patients with heart failure. A clinical issue is whether it is possible to select out a group of patients in whom benefit could be anticipated. Certainly that group might include patients with tachycardia, small hearts, myocardial ischaemia and hypertrophy. Two of the large recent studies [50, 51] (Table 12 and 13) suggest that there could be an advantage in dilated cardiomyopathy. The problem here is the extent to which the diagnosis of dilated cardiomyopathy has been truly established. The demonstration of a large heart with a uniform reduction of contraction is insufficient. A coronary angiogram is necessary. This has not been undertaken in the major studies. In MDC [50] the proportion of heart failure due to coronary heart disease was 0, in CIBIS [51] 55% and in the carvedilol studies [61] 48%. But these figures should be regarded with scepticism. In CIBIS the diagnosis of coronary heart disease was based on a history of coronary heart disease, previous myocardial infarction or a stenosis over 70%; 37% of patients had angina. In MDC the criterion for the exclusion of coronary heart disease was a stenosis less than 50%. It is unclear in these studies exactly how many patients underwent coronary angiography. Other work suggests that in such patients there is a very high incidence (about 45%) of severe three

Table 12. Metoprolol in dilated cardiomyopathy (MDC)

383 patients, EF < 40%, 12–18 months follow-up, upto 150 mg daily 73% male, 49 years, 93% in NYHA II or III, 82% on ACE,

	Placebo	Metoprolol	P
n	189	194	
Deaths	19	23	ns
Deaths/need for transplant	38	25	0.06
Discontinued Rx	31	23	ns
Increase of EF (%)	22 to 28	22 to 34	0.001
Heart rate	89 to 82	89 to 77	0.04
Exercise time	+15 s	+76 s	0.05

Quality of life improved in metoprolol group (P<0.01)

Lancet 1993; 342:1441–1446 [50].

Table 13. The cardiac insufficiency bisoprolol study (CIBIS)

641 patients, NYHA III or IV, Ef<40%, mean follow-up 1.9 years upto 5 mg daily, 60 years, 83% male, 36% IDCM, 90% on ACE, mean EF 25%

	Placebo	Bisoprolol	P
	321	320	
Deaths	67 (20.9%)	53 (16.6%)	ns
Withdrawals	82 (26%)	75 (23%)	ns
Heart failure with hospital admission	90	61	0.01
Deaths, no previous MI	42/187 (22.5%)	18/151 (12%)	0.01
Deaths, "IDCM"	23/115	11/117	0.01

Circulation 1994; 90:1765–1773 [51].

vessel coronary heart in patients previously thought to have idiopathic dilated cardiomyopathy [67, 68]. Furthermore the assessment of the significance of a coronary stenosis from the angiographic appearance is fraught and inaccurate.

Thus, the claim that in CIBIS the sub-group of patients with idiopathic dilated cardiomyopathy benefited in terms of mortality must be viewed with extreme caution. The data in MDC did not show any benefit in terms of mortality although there was a claim of benefit because of the combined endpoint of mortality and transplantation. The triallists were unfortunate that so many patients were referred for transplantation. The difficulty is that heart rate is one of many features that may determine the decision of the physician to refer the patient for transplantation. Furthermore physicians may have been able to detect whom was on β-blockade and may have had a bias against transplantation in that group. For these reasons a combined endpoint when dominated by transplantation is unsatisfactory.

There is an inevitable consequence from the previous arguments concerning the diagnosis of heart failure due to coronary heart disease and heart failure due to idiopathic dilated cardiomyopathy. Beta-blockers could be advantageous in heart failure because of their known benefits in patients with hypertension and angina. Many physicians do not use β-blockade as a treatment for heart failure but nevertheless are surprised by the large number of patients who are on β-blockers and at the same time on diuretics or ACE inhibitors. This comes about because these drugs are used for the treatment of angina and hypertension and since those conditions are frequently associated with heart failure the combination is also common. The argument can be taken further. If a patient has an established myocardial infarct then the treatment is aimed at optimising the situation with regard to the remaining viable tissue. By contrast if a patient has a non-Q wave infarct or severe myocardial ischaemia then treatment is related not just to the normal myocardium but to the diseased myocardium. An anti-ischaemic drug used in this context would paradoxically provide benefit in those patients without the major hallmark of coronary heart disease, namely previous myocardial infarction. In MDC, CIBIS and studies with other drugs such as calcium antagonists [69] the claimed benefit in patients with idiopathic dilated cardiomyopathy may be the consequence of wrong diagnosis and the subtle selection of just those patients who may benefit most from the known pharmacology of β-blockade.

Even if the on-going studies are positive one interpretation could be that the advantage is because the drugs are used to advantage in the treatment of known conditions, namely angina and hypertension, in patients with heart failure rather than for the treatment of heart failure itself. This distinction is crucial. In CIBIS 37% of patients had angina. Little is known about the effect of long-term β-blockade on mortality of patients with angina. Most of the evidence derives from patients who have sustained myocardial infarction.

Many of the above arguments apply equally to the analysis of the results of recent trials in terms of the relief symptoms. That has been a disappointing area for research workers in heart failure. A summary of some of the results is given in Table 6. The uniform finding is an increase in the ejection fraction. Exercise capacity in general has not been shown to improve in contrast to the results with other treatments such as ACE inhibitors [70]. New York Heart Association (NYHA) classification improved in the majority of the trials. Hospitalisation and mortality were variable. Many studies used a combined endpoint in order to increase power, for example the ANZ study (Table 14). The same problems

Table 14. Carvedilol in heart failure – The Australia/New Zealand trial

- 415 patients NYHA I (29%), II (59%) or III, EF < 45%, 88% previous myocardial infarct
  Carvedilol 25 mg bd. 27 withdrawals during 3 weeks or open Rx. Average of 19 months

- EF increased. EDD & ESD decreased. HR decreased by 6.8 bpm.

- No change in NYHA, SAS score, exercise duration, 6 min walk test

	Carvedilol	Placebo	
All deaths	20	26	0.76 (0.42–1.36)
All hospital admissions	99	120	0.77 (0.59–1.00)
Either of above	104	131	0.74 (0.57–0.95), P<0.02
Worsening heart failure	82	75	1.12 (0.82–1.53)

Australian/New Zealand Heart Failure Research Collaborative Group. Lancet 1997; 349:375–380 [59, 60].

arise as with the consideration overall mortality. Between 0% and 10% of patients were excluded in a test period biasing the trial in favour of the β-blocker. A sensitivity analysis would render many of the findings not significant. The largest single study, the ANZ study (Table 14), found no improvement in NYHA classification, SAS score for quality of life, exercise duration, 6 minute walking test or hospitalisation. Further the acceptance of hospitalisation as a measure of benefit to patients is not established. Hospitalisation depends critically on health resources, social circumstances, health delivery systems, financial gain and clinical circumstances. Hospitalisation may vary from the trivial to the crucial. Marginal benefit based on this endpoint needs careful examination.

The treatment of heart failure is now complex and the number of drugs available to the physician is large. Efforts should be made to avoid polypharmacy. For heart failure the standard treatment is diuretics and ACE inhibitors with or without digoxin. A β-blocker would be a fourth drug. In patients with coronary heart disease aspirin and a statin are probable drugs. Multiple drug usage is only too easy to achieve with the inevitable problems of drug interactions.

Conclusions

There is at present enthusiasm for the use of β-blockers in heart failure. The evidence lags far behind the enthusiasm. Undoubtedly there are selected patients in whom β-blockers are advantageous because of their known effects on angina pectoris and hypertension, which commonly accompany heart failure. Whether these drugs do have unequivocal long term benefits in terms of mortality and hospitalisation is not yet established because the trials have been over too short a period of time and with too small numbers of clinical events. The current trials will provide the definitive answer. For the present β-blockers should not be regarded as a necessary or essential part of the treatment of heart failure. On the other hand the reported trials provide considerable comfort for the use of β-blockers for angina or hypertension in patients who also have heart failure. Beta-blockade can be used in heart failure but not necessarily for heart failure. Physicians who understand the risks and benefits of such treatment in individual patients should use the drug carefully in sub-sets of patients.

References

1. Withering W (1785) An account of the foxglove, and some of its medical uses: with practical remarks on dropsy, and other diseases. London: GJJ and J Robinson
2. Slater JDH, Nabarro JDN (1958) Clinical experience with chlorothiazide. Lancet 1:124–126
3. The SOLVD Investigators (1991) Effect of enalapril on survival in patients with reduced left ventricular ejection fractions and congestive heart failure. N Engl J Med 325:293–302
4. The SOLVD investigators (1992) Effect of enalapril on mortality and the development of heart failure in asymptomatic patients with reduced left ventricular ejection fractions. N Engl J Med 327:685–691
5. Cohn JN, Johnson G, Ziesche S, Cobb F, Francis GS, Tristani F, Smith R, Dunkman WB, Loeb H, Wong M, Bhat G, Goldman S, Fletcher RD, Doherty J, Hughes CV, Carson P, Cintron G, Shabetai R, Haakenson C (1991) A comparison of enalapril with hydralazine-isosorbide dinitrate in the treatment of chronic congestive heart failure. N Engl J Med 325:302–310
6. Poole-Wilson PA, Robinson K (1989) Digoxin – a redundant drug in the treatment of congestive heart failure. Cardiovasc Drugs Ther 2:733–741

7. Jaeschke R, Oxman AD, Guyatt GH (1990) To what extent do congestive heart failure patients in sinus rhythm benefit from digoxin therapy? A systematic overview and meta-analysis. Am J Med 88:279–286
8. Kraus F, Rudolph C, Rudolph W (1993) Effectivity of digitalis in patients with chronic heart failure and sinus rhythm: an over view of randomised double-blind placebo-controlled studies. Herz 18:95–117
9. The Digitalis Investigation Group (1997) The effect of digoxin on mortality and morbidity in patients with heart failure. N Engl J Med 336:525–533
10. Poole-Wilson PA (1989) Chronic heart failure: cause, pathophysiology, prognosis, clinical manifestations, investigations. In: Julian DG, Camm AJ, Fox KF, Hall RJC, Poole-Wilson PA (eds.) Diseases of the Heart. London: Balliere-Tindall, S 24–36
11. Anand IS, Ferrari R, Kalra GS, Wahi PL, Poole-Wilson PA, Harris PC (1989) Edema of cardiac origin. Studies of body water and sodium, renal function, hemodynamic indexes, and plasma hormones in untreated congestive cardiac failure. Circulation 80:299–305
12. Anand IS, Veall N, Kalra GS, Ferrari R, Sutton G, Lipkin D, Harris P, Poole-Wilson PA (1989) Treatment of heart failure with diuretics: body compartments, renal function and plasma hormones. Eur Heart J 10:445–450.
13. Lipkin DP, Poole-Wilson PA (1986) Symptoms limiting exercise in chronic heart failure. Br Med J 292:1030–1031
14. Poole-Wilson PA (1993) Relation of pathophysiologic mechanisms to outcome in heart failure. J Am Coll Cardiol 22(Suppl A):22–29
15. Clark AL, Poole-Wilson PA, Coats AJS (1996) Exercise limitation in chronic heart failure: central role of the periphery. J Am Coll Cardiol 28:1092–1102
16. Harrington D, Anker SD, Chua TP, Webb-Peploe KM, Ponikowski PP, Poole-Wilson PA, Coats AJS (1997) Skeletal muscle function and its relation to exercise tolerance in chronic heart failure. J Am Coll Cardiol 30:1758–1764
17. Poole-Wilson PA, Ferrari R (1996) Role of skeletal muscle in the syndrome of chronic heart failure. [Review] [120 refs]. J Mol Cell Cardiol 28:2275–2285
18. Bayliss J, Norell M, Canepa-Anson R, Sutton G, Poole-Wilson P (1987) Untreated heart failure: clinical and neuroendocrine effects of introducing diuretics. Br Heart J 57:17–22
19. Remes J, Tikkanen I, Fyhrquist F, Pyorala K (1991) Neuroendocrine activity in untreated heart failure. Br Heart J 65:249–255
20. Narula J, Haider N, Virmani R, DiSalvo TG, Kolodgie FD, Hajjar RJ, Schmidt U, Semigran MJ, Dec GW, Khaw BA (1996) Apoptosis in myocytes in end-stage heart failure. N Engl J Med 335:1182–1189
21. Olivetti G, Abbi R, Quaini F, Kajstura J, Cheng W, Nitahara JA, Quaini, Di Loreto C, Beltrami CA, Krajewski S, Reed JC, Anversa P (1997) Apoptosis in the failing human heart. N Engl J Med 336:1131–1141

22. Anker SD, Chua TP, Ponikowski P, Harrington D, Swan JW, Kox WJ, Poole-Wilson PA, Coats AJS (1997) Hormonal Changes and Catabolic/Anabolic Imbalance in Chronic Heart Failure and Their Importance for Cardiac Cachexia. Circulation 96:526–534

23. Anker SD, Egerer KR, Volk HD, Kox WJ, Poole-Wilson PA, Coats AJ (1997) Elevated soluble CD14 receptors and altered cytokines in chronic heart failure. Am J Cardiol 79:1426–1430

24. Del Monte F, Kaumann AJ, Poole-Wilson PA, Wynne DG, Pepper J, Harding SE (1993) Coexistence of functioning β_1- and β_2-adrenoceptors in single myocytes from human ventricle. Circulation 88:854–863

25. Chidsey CA, Harrison DC, Braunwald E (1962) Augmentation of the plasma norepinephrine response to exercise in patients with congestive heart failure. N Engl J Med 267:650–654

26. Thomas JA, Marks BH (1978) Plasma norepinephrine in congestive heart failure. Am J Cardiol 1:233–243

27. Leimbach WNJ, Wallin BG, Victor RG, Aylward PE, Sundlof G, Mark AL (1986) Direct evidence from intraneural recordings for increased central sympathetic outflow in patients with heart failure. Circulation 73:913–919

28. Chidsey CA, Braunwald E, Morrow AG, Mason DT (1963) Myocardial norepinephrine concentration in man: effects of reserpine and of congestive heart failure. N Engl J Med 269:653–658

29. Petch MC, Nayler WG (1979 Concentration of catecholamines in human cardiac muscle. Br Heart J 41:340–344

30. Pierpont GL, Francis GS, DeMaster EG, Olivari MT, Ring WS, Goldenberg IF, Reynolds S, Cohn JN (1987) Heterogeneous myocardial catecholamine concentrations in patients with congestive heart failure. Am J Cardiol 60:316–321

31. Sole MJ, Helke CJ, Jacobowitz DM (1982) Increased dopamine in the failing hamster heart: transvesicular transport of dopamine limits the rate of norepinephrine synthesis. Am J Cardiol 49:1682–1690

32. Bohm M, La Rosee K, Schwinger RH, Erdmann E (1995) Evidence for reduction of norepinephrine uptake sites in the failing human heart. J Am Coll Cardiol 25:146–153

33. Kingwell B, Thompson J, Kaye D, McPherson A, Jennings G, Esler M (1994) Heart rate spectral analysis, cardiac norepinephine spillover, and muscle sympathetic nerve activity during human sympathetic nervous activation and failure. Circulation 90:234–240

34. Kaye DM, Lambert GW, Lefkovits J, Morris M, Jennings G, Esler MD (1994) Neurochemical evidence of cardiac sympathetic activation and increased central nervous system norepinephrine turnover in severe congestion. J Am Coll Cardiol 23:570–578

35. Bristow MR, Ginsburg R, Minobe W, Cubicciotti RS, Sageman WS, Lurie K, Billingham ME, Harrison DC, Stinson EB (1982) Decreased catecholamine sensitivity and β-adrenergic-receptor density in failing human hearts. N Engl J Med 307:205–211

36. Harding SE, Brown LA, Wynne DG, Davies CH, Poole-Wilson PA (1994) Mechanism of β adrenoceptor desensitisation in the failing human heart. Cardiovasc Res 28:1451–1460

37. Banner NR, Patel N, Cox AP, Patton HE, Lachno DR, Yacoub MH (1989) Altered sympathoadrenal response to dynamic exercise in cardiac transplant recipients. Cardiovasc Res 23:965–972

38. Waagstein F, Hjalmarson A, Varauskas I (1975) Effect of chronic β-adrenergic receptor blockade in congestive cardiomyopathy. Br Heart J 37:1022–1036

39. Swedberg K, Hjalmarson A, Waagstein F, Wallentin I (1980) Beneficial effects of long-term β-blockade in congestive cardiomyopathy. Br Heart J 44:117–133

40. Heilbrunn SM, Shah P, Bristow MR, Valantine HA, Ginsburg R, Fowler MB (1989) Increased β-receptor density and improved hemodynamic response to catecholamine stimulation during long-term metoprolol therapy in heart failure from dilated cardiomyopathy. Circulation 79:483–490

41. Nemanich JW, Veith RC, Abrass IB, Stratton JR (1990) Effects of metoprolol on rest and exercise cardiac function and plasma catecholamines in chronic congestive heart failure secondary to ischemic or idiopathic cardiomyopathy. Am J Cardiol 66:843–848

42. Anderson JL, Gilbert EM, O'Connell JB, Renlund D, Yanowitz F, Murray M, Roskelley M, Mealey P, Volkman K, Deitchman D, Bristow M (1991) Long-term (2 year) beneficial effects of β-adrenergic blockade with bucindolol in patients with idiopathic dilated cardiomyopathy. J Am Coll Cardiol 17:1373–1381

43. Ikram H, Fitzpatrick D (1981) Double-blind trial of chronic oral β-blockade in congestive cardiomyopathy. Lancet 2:490–493

44. Currie PJ, Kelly MJ (1984) Oral β-adrenergic blockade with metroprolol in chronic severe dilated cardiomyopathy. J Am Coll Cardiol 3:203–209.

45. Leung WH, Lau CP, Wong CK, Cheng CH, Tai YT, Lim SP (1990) Improvement in exercise performance and hemodynamics by labetalol in patients with idiopathic dilated cardiomyopathy. Am Heart J 119:884–890

46. Engelmeier RS, O'Connell JB, Walsh R, Rad N, Scanlon PJ, Gunnar RM (1985) Improvement in symptoms and exercise tolerance by metoprolol in patients with dilated cardiomyopathy: a double-blind, randomised, placebo-controlled trial. Circulation 72:536–546

47. Anderson JL, Lutz JR, Gilbert EM, Sorensen SG, Yanowitz FG, Menlove RL, Bartholomew M (1985) A randomized trial of low-dose β-blockade therapy for idiopathic dilated cardiomyopathy. Am J Cardiol 55:471–475

48. The German and Austrian Xamoterol Study Group (1988) Double-blind placebo-controlled comparison of digoxin and xamoterol in chronic heart failure. Lancet 1:489–493

49. The Xamoterol in Severe Heart Failure Study Group (1990) Xamoterol in severe heart failure. Lancet 336:1–6

50. Waagstein F, Bristow MR, Swedberg K, Camerini F, Fowler MB, Silver MA, Gilbert EM, Johnson MR, Goss FG, Hjalmarson A (1993) Beneficial

effects of metoprolol in idiopathic dilated cardiomyopathy. Lancet 342:1441–46

51. CIBIS Investigators and Committees (1994) A randomized trial of β-blockade in heart failure. The Cardiac Insufficiency Bisoprolol Study (CIBIS). CIBIS Investigators and Committees. Circulation 90:1765–1773

52. Metra M, Nardi M, Giubbini R, Dei Cas L (1994) Effects of short- and long-term carvedilol administration on rest and exercise hemodynamic variables, exercise capacity and clinical conditions in patients with idiopathic dilated cardiomyopathy. J Am Coll Cardiol 24:1678–1687

53. Olsen SL, Gilbert EM, Renlund DG, Taylor DO, Yanowitz FD, Bristow MR (1995) Carvedilol improves left ventricular function and symptoms in chronic heart failure: a double-blind randomized study. J Am Coll Cardiol 25:1225–1231

54. Krum H, Sackner-Bernstein JD, Goldsmith RL, Kukin ML, Schwartz B, Penn J, Medina N, Yushak M, Horn E, Katz SD, et al. (1995) Double-blind, placebo-controlled study of the long-term efficacy of carvedilol in patients with severe chronic heart failure. Circulation 92:1499–1506

55. Bristow MR, Gilbert EM, Abraham WT, Adams KF, Fowler MB, Hershberger RE, Kubo SH, Narahara KA, Ingersoll H, Krueger S, Young S, Shusterman N (1996) Carvedilol produces dose-related improvements in left ventricular function and survival in subjects with chronic heart failure. MOCHA Investigators [comment]. Circulation 94:2807–2816

56. Colucci WS, Packer M, Bristow MR, Gilbert EM, Cohn JN, Fowler MB, Krueger SK, Hershberger R, Uretsky BF, Bowers JA, Sackner-Bernstein JD, Young ST, Holcslaw TL, Lukas MA (1996) Carvedilol inhibits clinical progression in patients with mild symptoms of heart failure. US Carvedilol Heart Failure Study Group. Circulation 94:2800–2806

57. Packer M, Colucci WS, Sackner-Bernstein JD, Liang CS, Goldscher DA, Freeman I, Kukin ML, Kinhal V, Udelson JE, Klapholz M, Gottlieb SS, Pearle D, Cody RJ, Gregory JJ, Kantrowitz NE, LeJemtel TH, Young ST, Lukas MA, Shusterman NH (1996) Double-blind, placebo-controlled study of the effects of carvedilol in patients with moderate to severe heart failure. The PRECISE Trial. Prospective Randomized Evaluation of Carvedilol on Symptoms and Exercise. Circulation 94:2793–2799

58. Cohn JN, Fowler MB, Bristow MR, Colucci WS, Gilbert EM, Kinhal V, Krueger SK, LeJemtel T, Narahara, KA, Packer M, Young ST, Holcslaw TL, Lukas MA (1997) Safety and efficacy of carvedilol in severe heart failure. The U.S. Carvedilol Heart Failure Study Group. J Cardiac Failure 3:173–179

59. Australia/New Zealand heart failure research collaborative group (1997) Randomised, placebo-controlled trial of carvedilol in patients with congestive heart failure due to ischaemic heart disease. Lancet 349:375–380

60. Anonymous (1995) Effects of carvedilol, a vasodilator-β-blocker, in patients with congestive heart failure due to ischemic heart disease. Australia-New Zealand Heart Failure Research Collaborative Group. Circulation 92:212–218

61. Packer M, Bristow MR, Cohn JN, Colucci WS, Fowler MB, Gilbert EM, Shusterman NH (1996) for the U.S. Carvedilol Heart Failure Study Group. The effect of carvedilol on morbidity and mortality in patients with chronic heart failure. N Engl J Med 334:1349–1355
62. Doughty RN, Sharpe N (1997) Beta-adrenergic blocking agents in the treatment of congestive heart failure: mechanisms and clinical results. Annual Review of Medicine 48:103–114
63. Doughty RN, Rodgers A, Sharpe N, MacMahon S (1997) Effects of β-blocker therapy on mortality in patients with heart failure. A systematic overview of randomized controlled trials. Eur Heart J 18:560–565
64. Heidenreich PA, Lee TT, Massie BM (1997) Effect of β-blockade on mortality in patients with heart failure: a meta-analysis of randomized clinical trials. J Am Coll Cardiol 30:27–34
65. Lechat P (1997) β-blocker treatment in heart failure. In: Puddu PE, Bing RJ, Campa PP, Poole-Wilson PA (eds.) Congestive Heart Failure. Rome: Cardioricerca, S 465–498
66. Cleland JGF, Bristow MR, Erdmann E, Remme WJ, Swedberg K, Waagstein F (1996) Beta-blocking agents in heart failure. Should they be used and how? Eur Heart J 17:1629–1639
67. Figulla HR, Kellerman AB, Stille-Siegener M, Heim A, Kreuzer H (1992) Significance of coronary angiography, left heart catheterisation, and endomyocardial biopsy for the diagnosis of idiopathic dilated cardiomyopathy. Am Heart J 124:1251–1257
68. Benton RE, Coughlin SS, Teft MC (1994) Predictors of coronary angiography in patients with idiopathic dilated cardiomyopathy: the Washington, DC Dilated Cardiomyopathy Study. J Clin Epidemiol 47:501–511
69. Poole-Wilson PA (!997) Amlodipine in chronic heart failure. N Engl J Med 336:1023
70. Townend JN, Littler WA (1993) Angiotensin converting enzyme inhibitors in heart failure: how good are they? Br Heart J 69:373–375

Case Reports

β-Receptor Blocker Therapy in Dilated Cardiomyopathy After Doxorubicine Therapy

A. Stäblein and D. Hartmann

History

A 31-year-old patient was admitted for further investigation to our outpatient clinic under the suspicion of having progressive renal insufficiency with marked edema of the legs. The patient reported exertional dyspnea after climbing two flights of stairs. Orthopnea was not present, and nyctura occurred maximally twice per night.

In the long-term history of the patient there was T-lymphoblastic acute leukemia diagnosed 5 years earlier and treated with vincirstine, doxorubicin, prednisolone and methotrexate intrathecally, cytosine-arabinoside intrathecally, and dexamethasone intrathecally, according to the BMFT-ALL/AUL protocol. Therapy was performed as induction treatment, consoliation therapy and maintenance therapy including radiation of the CNS and mediastinum. Maintenance therapy was continued for 2 years, with the patient in remission up to his admission to hospital.

The patient smoked 20–30 cigarrettes a day, had hyperlipidemia and arterial hypertension, but no history of diabetes mellitus; his father suffered from coronary heart disease. He admitted to casual drinking of beer in small amounts.

Physical Examination

The patient's general condition was slightly reduced with marked overweight (186 cm, 116 kg). There were no palpable lymphatic nodes and no inflammation of the throat; lungs were normal in auscultation and percussion. Heartbeat was regular without pathological murmurs, blood pressure at 190/120 mmHg, and the heart rat 120/min. The patient's belly soft and adipose; liver and spleen were not enlarged, not where the kidneys tender. There were no pathological abdominal resistances or pain. Massive, bilateral edema of the calf and peripheral pulses were palpable.

Laboratory Measurements

Electrolytes, liver enzymes and urea were within the normal ranges, creatinine concentration was 1.8 mg/dl, creatinine clearance 79 ml/min, uric acid concentration 9.8 mg/dl, total protein 61 g/l, albumin 49%, a_1- and a_2-globulin each 20%, γ-globulin 11%, cholesterol 174 mg/dl, HDL-cholesterol 25 mg/dl, and cholesterol/HDL-cholesterol 7.0. Slight granulocytosis (79%) with lymphopenia and eosinopenia (16% and 0%) respectively and normal absolute white blood cell count were registered. Thyroid hormones and TSH were within normal ranges. In the urine medium-degree erythrocyturia with little granulocyturia and proteinuria (154 mg albumin/g creatinine) was found, there were no bacteria in the urine.

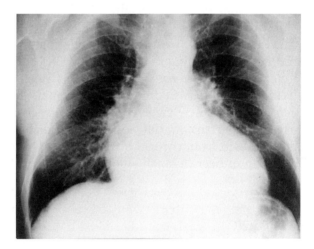

Fig. 1. Chest X-ray of the decompensated patient with right- and left heart dilatation, central venous and pulmonary venous congestion, and signs of pulmonary hypertension

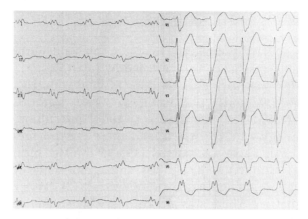

Fig. 2. Resting ECG of the Decompensated patient

Values for anticytoplasmic antibodies, the anti-DNA, antinucleic antibodies, cryoglobulins and anti-streptolysine were normal. There were no significantly elevated antibody concentrations for Coxsackie-, echo-, influenza-, parainfluenza-, adeno- or cytomegaly viruses

The chest X-ray in Fig. 1 showed a bilaterally enlarged heart with signs of central venous and pulmonary venous congestion. Prominent pulmonary hili and peripheral rarefication of pulmonary arteries consistent with pulmonary arterial hypertension were apparent. There was no sign of infiltration or pleural effusion.

As shown by the ECG in Fig. 2, sinus tachycardia was 103/min, and there was complete left bundle branch block with concomitant disturbances of repolarisation.

Echocardiography

Echocardiography revealed a significantly enlarged left atrium (60 mm) and an enlarged left ventricle with severely reduced contraction in a diffuse pattern (EDD 64 mm, FS 10%). The right heart was of normal size. There was slight mitral regurgitation, but no signs of valvular disease.

Heart Catheterization

Slight postcapillary pulmonary hypertension with normal pulmonary arteriolar resistance was revealed by heart catherization. The cardiac index was severely reduced (PCW 20 mmHg, PA 35/18 mmHg, RV 35/9 mmHg, RA 9mmHg, CO 4.1 l/min, Cl 1.7 l/m^2 kgKG). Increased left ventricular systolic and filling pressures (195/18 mmHg) were registered, and there was no pressure drop when the aortic valve was passed (195/95 mmHg, mean pressure 130 mmHg). The left ventricle was angiographically dilated with severe reduction of contraction (EDV 320 ml, EF 32%), but no mitral regurgitation. There was no coronary macroangiopathy. Five endomyocardial biopsies were taken from the right ventricular septum.

Histological Examination of Endomyocardial Biopsies

Histological examination of endomyocardial biopsies revealed slightly hypertrophied myocardial cells without signs of inflammatory infiltration or myocarditis.

Abdominal Ultrasound

Abdominal ultrasound showed slight hepatomegaly with normal structure and slight splenomegaly. Kidneys were of normal size and morphology and without signs of postrenal obstruction.

Pulmonary Function Test

Pulmonary function test revealed normal spirometry (Vc$_{max}$ 4.5 l, FEV$_1$ 3.6 l, normal resistance) and slight hypoxia with normal ventilation (pO$_2$ 76 mmHg, pCO$_2$ 39.7 mmHg, pH 7.40).

Radionuclide Ventriculography

At rest, left ventricular function was significantly reduced without increase under exercise conditions (EF 29% vs. 28%), as shown by radionuclide ventriculography.

Diagnosis

Diagnosis of the patient was as follows:

- Dilated cardiomyopathy due to chronic arterial hypertension after cardiac damage with doxorubicin chemotherapy.
- Chronically compensated renal insufficiency.
- Arterial hypertension.
- Complete remission 5 years ater T-lymphoblastic acute leukemia.
- Hyperuricemia.

Follow-up

Initially the patient was treated with the standard therapy for left ventricular failure (20 mg enalapril bid, 0.1 mg digitoxin, 50 mg hydrochlorothiazide). After recompensation and with severely compromised left ventricular function, therapy with 6.25 mg carvedilol bid was started, which the patient tolerated well. β-blocker dosage was doubled after 2 and 4 weeks, respectively reaching a final dosage of 25 mg carvedilol bid, which was tolerated without adverse events. The patient felt well and was without signs of cardiac decompensation. After 2 months cardiac function was nearly normal so that the patient returned to work and was able to climb three flights of stairs at normal speed without dyspnea.

ECG (After Therapy)

ECG after therapy revealed a sinus rhythm of 74/min and complete left bundle-branch block with concomitant disturbances of repolarization.

Exercise Tolerance Test (After Therapy)

In the exercise tolerance test following therapy, exercise at 100 W, was interrupted after 7 min because of fatigue, but there was no inadequate dyspnea or angina pectoris. Blood pressure profile was normal (135/85 mmHg, 76/min at rest, 165/90 mmHg, 120/min at submaximal exercise) with fast recovery within 4 min.

Echocardiography (After Therapy)

Left atrium and ventricle were normal-sized, and left ventricular contraction slightly compromised without segmental abnormalities (LVEDD 56 mm, FS 28%), as shown by echocardiography following therapy. Right atrium and ventricle were normal, and there were no signs of mitral regurgitation or valvular disease.

Radionuclide Ventriculography (After Therapy)

In radionuclide ventriculography following therapy, ejection fraction was slightly reduced at rest with adequate increase under bicycle exercise at 75 W (43% to 51%). Improvement was significant compared to the results before β-blocker treatment.

Chest X-ray (After Therapy)

As shown by the chest X-ray in Fig. 3, the left heart was slightly enlarged after therapy, but there were no signs of central venous or pulmonary venous congestion, there was no infiltration or pleural effusion.

Discussion

The patient described above showed global decompensation of heart function 5 years after systemic chemotherapy with doxorubicin. After exclusion of coronary heart disease and histological examina-

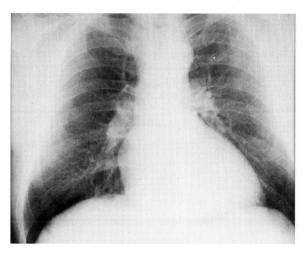

Fig. 3. Chest X-ray of the recompensated patient with only slight left heart dilatation, but no signs of central venous or pulmonary venous congestion or pulmonary hypertension

tion without signs of myocarditis, this must be interpreted as hypertensive cardiomyopathy after additional toxic myocardial damage.

After initiation of standard medical therapy using digitoxin, diuretics and ACE inhibitors, sinus tachycardia was still present even after recompensation. We started uptitration of carvedilol with 6.25 mg bid and were able to double the dose every 2 weeks without adverse events up to 25 mg carvedilol bid. Under chronic therapy, symptoms at rest disappeared and exercise tolerance normalized with improvement of left ventricular ejection fraction to nearly normal values. Hyperuricemia was treated successfully with allopurinol (100 mg/die), and blood cell count did not change in follow-up investigations. The patient showed a normal resting heart rate and a normal heart-rate response under stress conditions, implicating a normalized neurohumoral balance. Parameters of left ventricular function (echocardiography, radionuclide ventriculography) returned to nearly normal values in accordance with the results of the trials performed with carvedilol in patients with moderate to severe heart failure, in whom a significant improvement of ejection fraction and symptom atology could be seen [1, 2]. Our patient was able to return to his fromer profession under continued medication.

References

1. Packer M, Colucci WS, Sackner-Bernstein JD et al (1996) Double-blind, placebo controlled study of carvedilol in patients with moderate to severe heart failure. The PRECISE trial. Circulation 94:2793–2799
2. Bristow MR, Gilbert EM, Abraham WT et al (1995) Multicenter oral carvedilol heart failure assessment (MOCHA): a six month dose-response evaluation in class II-IV patients. Circulation 92(Suppl I):142

β-Blocker Therapy in Severe Cardiac Heart Failure

D. Hartmann and A. Stäblein

History

A 52-years-old man reported progressive dyspnoea of more than 4 months. He could not walk more than 200 m and he was hospitalized due to worsening heart failure 2 weeks prior to examination. He was treated with an ACE inhibitor and a loop-active diuretic (furosemide 40 mg, captopril 12.5 mg). After demission he was admitted to our outpatient clinic in order to discuss the indication for elective cardiac transplant. Other relevant diseases in the past were not reported. The patient smoked 15 cigarrettes per day; drinking of alcohol was not permitted.

Physical Examination

The patient was in a rather normal general condition and had normal weight (173 cm/70 kg). Blood pressure was 92/63 mmHg and heart rate 114/min; heartbeat was regular. There were rales over both lungs. Furthermore, there was bilateral edema of the legs, and the liver was slightly enlarged.

Technical Findings

The ECG showed a sinus tachycardia (123/min) and a complete left bundle brunch block with typically disturbed repolarization. Echocardiographically we found an enlarged left atrium (48 mm) and left ventricle (66 mm end-diastolic) with a diffuse distur-

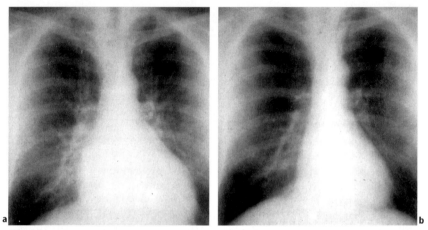

Fig. 1.

bance of contractility. In radionuclide ventriculography, the ejection fraction at rest was 11%. Maximal oxygen consumption was severely reduced to 11 ml/kg min. The laboratory measurements showed slight hyperglycemia (134 mg%) and pathological liver enzymes (SGOT 35 u/l, SGPT 43 u/l). The chest X-ray showed a significantly enlarged heart with signs of pulmonary venous congestion. Heart dimension ratio was 0.54 (Fig. 1a). Angiographically a coronary macroangiopathy could be excluded. As a result, dilated cardiomyopathy was diagnosed.

Follow-up

The findings of the examination fulfilled all criteria for including the patient in the elective cardiac transplant program, but this therapeutic option was refused by the patient. After cardiac recompensation by treatment with the standard therapy of chronic heart failure (0.07 mg digitoxin, 150 mg captopril, 40 mg torasemide and 50 mg spironolactone per day) as well as anticoagulation with phenprocoumon, we started an additional therapy with carvedilol. The initial dose was 3.125 mg twice a day, with the patient reporting fatigue and dizziness. Two weeks later the patient felt well, and in the following 4 weeks we titrated carvedilol up to 2×12.5 mg. At this time the patient had to be hospitalized because of severe hypotension (RR 70/35 mmHg) with acute prerenal failure (creatinine 5.7 mg%). The therapy with carvedilol was stopped immediately and ACE inhibitor was reduced to 12.5 mg captopril per day. Under substitution of volume the patient soon regained a stable cardiopulmonary condition, and creatinine could be normalized within a few days. In the following weeks ACE inhibitor could be titrated up to a dose of 150 mg captopril daily. Three months later we again tried an additional therapy with carvedilol, but during this trial titration time was prolonged. Within 6 months we reached the target dose of 2×25 mg carvedilol, which was now very well tolerated by the patient. His physical condition was much better than 6 months ago, and he was able to ascend two flights of stairs without dyspnea. Physical examination showed a significant rise in blood pressure (120/80 mmHg) and reduction of heart rate (68/min), and there were no longer any signs of cardiac decompensation. Echocardiographically the left atrium now had a normal size (39 mm), whereas the left ventricle was just as enlarged as before (68 mm end-diastolic). However left ventricular function was significantly improved, as shown by radionuclide ventriculography (EF 28%). The chest X-ray no longer showed signs of pulmonary venous congestion, and the heart thoracic quotient was now in a normal range (HTQ 0.46); (Fig. 1b). Peak oxygen consumption was also improved (14.8 ml/kg min) in cardio-pulmonary exercise testing. Although the results of examinations showed a significant improvement in left ventricular function, the therapeutic option for elective cardiac transplant still existed. Under the aspect of quality of life the patient refused the inclusion into a transplant program.

Discussion

The patient described above had dilated cardiomyopathy with severe reduction of left ventricular function (NYHA III). Angiographically coronary heart disease could be excluded. Moreover, there were no signs of metabolic or hypertensive disorders as pathophysiological reasons for left ventricular dysfunction.

The prognosis of untreated chronic heart failure is bad. The CONSENSUS trial showed a 1-year mortality rate of 52% for patients with end-stage heart failure [12].

The standard therapy of chronic heart failure consists of ACE inhibitors, diuretics and glycosides. The results of the CONSEN-SUS trial [12] and SOLVD trials [15] underlined the improvement in survival in patients with severe heart failure treated with ACE inhibitors.

In order to reach an improvement in mortality, it is important to achieve a target dose of 150 mg captopril or 20 mg enalapril per day. Additionally, therapy with glycosides is an established procedure and is able to improve clinical symptoms of heart failure; nevertheless, the DIG trial showed no significant improvement in mortality [13].

Recently several trials examined the effect of β-adrenergic blocking agents, which consistently improve left ventricular function in subjects with chronic heart failure [6, 10, 16–18]. An improvement in survival in patients with chronic heart failure was seen in the meta-analysis of several trials with carvedilol [14].

Conclusion

Patients with chronic heart failure should be treated with β-blockers in addition to the standard therapy consisting of ACE inhibitors, diuretics and glycosides [1–7, 16–18]. Carvedilol, a β-blocker with vasodilator effects, was shown to ameliorate symptoms, diminish disability, and reduce the morbidity associated with moderate to severe heart failure independent of the cause of the disorder [13–14]. It seems to be very important to titrate carvedilol very slowly up to the target dose of 2×25 mg after having established standard therapy of heart failure at sufficient doses. Nevertheless, there may be adverse events, as we have seen in our case report described above. An adjustment in concomitant therapy may not require general withdrawal from carvedilol. In our case the patient was again treated with carvedilol, and about 1 year later we saw a significant improvement in ejection fraction and physical condition.

References

1. Asseman P, McFadden E, Bauchart JJ, Loybeyre C, Thery C (1994) Who do beta-blockers help in idiopathic dilated cardiomyopathy-frequency mismatch? Lancet 344:803–804
2. Böhm M, Beuckelmann D, Brown L et al (1988a) Reduction of beta adrenoceptor density and evaluation of positive inotropic responses in isolated, diseased human myocardium. Eur Heart J 9:844–852
3. Böhm M, La Rosee K, Schwinger RHG, Erdmann E (1995) Evidence for reduction of norepinephrine uptake sites in the failing human heart. J Am Coll Cardiol 25:146–153
4. Bristow MR, Ginsberg W, Minobe RS (1982) Decreased catecholamine sensitivity and beta-adrenergic-receptor density in failing human hearts. N Engl J Med 307:205–211
5. CIBIS Investigators and Committees (1994) A randomized trial of β-blockade in heart failure: the Cardiac Insufficiency Bisoprolol Study (CIBIS). Circulation 90:1765–1773
6. Cohn JN, Archibald DG, Olivari MT et al (1984) Plasma norepinephrine as a guide to prognosis in patients with chronic congestive heart failure. N Engl J Med 311:819–823
7. The CONSENSUS Trial Study Group (1987) Effects of Enalapril on mortality in severe congestive heart failure: results of the Cooperative North Scandinavian Enalapril Survival Study (CONSENSUS). N Engl J Med 316:1429–1435
8. DIG, Digitalis Investigation Group, Gorlin R et al (1997) N Engl J Med 336, 525
9. Doughery RN, MacMagon S, Sharpe N (1994) Beta-blockers in heart failure: promising or proved? J A Coll Cardiol 23:814–821
10. Heilbrunn SM, Shah P, Valentine HA et al (1986) Increased beta-receptor density and improved hemodynamic response to catecholamine stimulation during chronic metoprolol therapy. Circulation 74 (Suppl II):II–310
11. Held P (1993) Effects of beta blockers on ventricular dysfunction after myocardial function: tolerability and survival effects. Am J Cardiol 71:39c–44c
12. Packer M (1990) Pathophysiological mechanisms underlying the effect of β-adrenergic agonists and antagonists on functional capacity and survival in chronic heart failure. Circulation 82 (Suppl I):I77–I88
13. Packer M et al (1996) The effect of Carvedilol on morbidity and mortality in patients with chronic heart failure. N Engl J Med 334:1349–1355
14. The SOLVD Investigators (1991) Effects of enalapril on survival in patients with reduced left ventricular ejection fractions and congestive heart failure. N Engl J Med 325:293–302
15. Waagstein F (1995) β-blockers in congestive heart failure due to idiopathic dilated cardiomyopathy. Curr Opin Cardiol 10:322–331

16. Waagstein F, Hjalmarson Å, Varnauskas E, Wallentin I (1980) Effect of chronic beta-adrenergic receptor blockade in congestive cardiomyopathy. Br Heart J 44:117
17. Waagstein F, Caidahl K, Wallentin I, Bergh CH, Hjalmarson Å (1989) Long-term beta-blockade in congestive cardiomyopathy: effects of acute and chronic metoprolol treatment followed by withdrawal and readministration of metoprolol. Circulation 80:551–563

Subject Index

Printing and binding: Druckerei Triltsch, Würzburg